Oneness

The Simple
Self-Healing Secret
You Were Never
Supposed to Know

LD Chen & MeiMei Fox

LD Chen & MeiMei Fox

ONENESS:
The Simple Self-Healing Secret You were Never Supposed to Know

Cover Design | Jared Oriel
Editor | Laura Yorke

Disclaimer

You can't find another practice as effective, as direct, yet as simple as Oneness.
– Grandmaster Yu Hongkun

DEDICATION

Nine years ago, a Chinese book about Oneness set me on the path to healing – and utterly transformed my life.

I dedicate this book to you, dear reader, because my most profound hope is that it will do the same for you.

LD Chen
San Francisco, CA

CONTENTS

Part IV: The Practice of Oneness

Part V: The Life of Oneness

Prologue

What Is Oneness?

When I was 32, I was suffering deeply—
from a heart attack, asthma, anxiety, burnout,
liver disease, back pain, neck stiffness,
and numbness in my left leg.

For the next ten years, I hunted constantly for treatments.
I visited famous doctors across numerous cities.
I tried modern medicine, Chinese medicine.
Tai Chi, physical therapy, swimming… everything.
Nothing worked.
I almost gave up.

Then one day, my Tai Chi teacher told me about **Oneness**.
I decided to give it a try.
I bought more than 20 books about the practice and
read them all.

And then—there was one.
When I read it for the first time, I felt something.
The author later became my sensei:
Grandmaster Yu Hongkun.
At that time, I thought Oneness was just for healing.

ONENESS

Because Grandmaster Yu is a Kung Fu master,
my first impression of Oneness was simple:
Kung Fu and healing. That's it.
Even though the book included so much more.
I wasn't sure it would actually work.

Honestly, I still believed hospitals and medicine
were the only "scientific" way.
But I began to practice.
Slowly, my symptoms began to disappear.

I became a disciple of Mr. Yu.
I listened to his teachings.
I practiced more.
I read his book again—a second time.
A third time.
I kept practicing…
One year.
Two years.
Nine years.

And Oneness kept opening up for me.
It became something much, much more vast
than just healing.
It became something I never expected,
a transformative practice.
It kept surprising me.
Sometimes I would pause and look at
the new LD emerging—
a different person.
And then… a different one again.

I thought:
Oneness is not just about healing.
It's not just about Kung Fu.

There's so much more.
It's life-changing.
And no—not like the "life-changing" people often throw around.
This is different.
 Trust me, I get the doubt.
I was there, too.
In fact, at the beginning, I even doubted whether
it could help me heal,
let alone change my life.

But Oneness is something that can completely
transform a person
from the inside out,
layer by layer,
deeper and deeper.
It is limitless.

I know so many people today are looking for healing.
Maybe you suffer from a chronic illness.
Maybe you're struggling with your mental health.
Maybe—like me—you've already tried everything:
doctors, medications, techniques, teachings...
but nothing has helped.

So yes—when you're suffering,
healing is the only thing you can focus on.
I understand.
I was there, too.
When you suffer every single day—
it's real.
You feel it.
You live inside it.
And the biggest question becomes:
How do I make this pain go away?

ONENESS

Because when your body hurts all day long,
How can you even think about happiness?
How can you think about helping others?
When someone is buried in depression—
Sometimes they can't even get through daily tasks.
They don't have the energy to take care of themselves,
let alone their family, their partner, or their kids.
It's not that they don't care.
It's that their body and mind sim-
ply can't carry that weight anymore.

So yes—
at the beginning, it *is* just about healing.
And let me say it clearly:
Oneness can heal.
For sure, it can heal.

But then—
people ask me,
"I heard Oneness can clear your mind,
help you make better decisions, even bring wisdom.
Is that true?"
And I say:
Yes. Absolutely.

But most people never get there—
because they stop once the healing begins.
And that's okay.

It's like climbing a mountain.
At first, it's hard.
Your view does not change.
Even though you're putting in such effort.
But the moment you take that first step,
you begin to rise.

And eventually—after a while—
you stop and look back.
And suddenly:

The view has changed.
It has become broader.
It has become more beautiful.
That's what happens inside you when you begin to practice
Oneness.
You begin to feel better.
Your mind begins to clear.
You get less angry, or maybe you can hold the tension more gently.
You feel lighter.
The view inside starts to shift.

Some people don't even notice it's happening.
But if you keep climbing—
the view keeps getting better.
And one day, you realize:
All your symptoms are gone.
And something even deeper inside you has changed.
You feel more empathy.
More love.
Your anger? Almost gone.
And your family sees it, too.

You have reached the halfway point.
And it's beautiful.
You may choose to stop here.
Enjoy the view.
Already it's a wonderful life.
Isn't it?

But a few people—
just a few—
they want to go higher.
What's at the top of the mountain? they ask.
So they keep climbing.
Keep exploring.
And as they do, their whole body begins to shift—
layer by layer.
They become newer.
Freer.
And then… new benefits begin to arrive.
Beauty they never expected.
Views they never imagined.
They find themselves thinking:
How can life be this beautiful?
How can a person live with so little burden,
so little Self—yet so much joy?

And here's the funny part—
when you climb a physical mountain, there is a limit.
There's a top.
But with Oneness, there's no top.
No limit.
It's endless.
The more you explore,
the more you discover.
And if I told you how beautiful those views are—
you might not believe me.
But those who practice Oneness…
they know.
There's a reason they keep going.

When I look back now,
I feel so grateful.

The years of suffering…
the illnesses I battled…
they didn't just bring me pain.
They brought me a gift.
They gave me a life
I never could have imagined.

If you're suffering right now,
maybe your pain is your gift, too.
Your tipping point.
Don't waste it.
Don't blame fate.
The doorway to wisdom is opening for you.
Now, maybe you understand
why I speak so much about it,
why I am so eager to explain people what Oneness is.
And yet even now—
I still can't explain it fully.

I'm reminded of the first chapter of the *Tao Te Ching*:

> *The Tao that can be told is not the eternal Tao.*
> *The name that can be named is not the eternal name.*
> *The nameless is the origin of heaven and earth.*

Many people ask me, *What is Oneness?*
And for over a year, I've tried to find a way to explain it clearly.
Grandmaster Yu gave me only one instruction:
"Remember, LD—stay with the true Oneness.
Don't make Oneness small just to fit the trends."

Some advisors helping me with this book and the Oneness
Institute have said,
"This won't work.
If you want to market this,

ONENESS

you must focus on one disease—
like depression, anxiety, or chronic back pain…"
But I received a different message.

Early on the morning of April 25, 2025,
while visiting my coauthor in Honolulu,
and staying at a hotel in Waikiki,
I awoke early and began my morning practice.
This entire message flowed out of me—naturally.
I wrote it down just as it came.

So…
If you suffer from chronic disease,
If you struggle with your mental health,
If you want a clearer mind or better decision-making,
If you want to heal your relationships,
If you feel lost, unhappy, or unsure why you're even here...
If you're searching for something more—

Welcome to Oneness.

INTRODUCTION

From Skeptic to Sensei

This practice is much simpler than you can imagine.
This practice is much more powerful than you can imagine.

What if the key to physical healing, emotional stability, mental clarity, and effortless energy has been within you all along, but you were never taught how to access it?

What if the reason you feel exhausted, restless, stuck, or burnt out isn't because life is too stressful, but because you're constantly fighting against your own natural power?

What if everything you've been searching for—health, peace, happiness, connection—isn't something you must battle endlessly to achieve, but rather something you need only remember?

This is what Oneness is all about.

Oneness is not a philosophy you must analyze, a complex technique you must master, or a belief system you must adopt. It's not another item to add to your already packed to-do list. It doesn't demand that you spend a great deal of your hard-earned money. It does not require you to break yet another bad habit.

It's something far simpler. Something so simple, in fact, that most people overlook it.

Oneness is about *being*. The direct, physical experience of just being.

And it isn't something you do only during practice. It applies to your whole life—your relationships, your work, your business, and your decision-making. There is no limit to what you can experience.

My Healing Journey to Oneness

At age 32, I had everything the world told me I should want.

I was the founder and CEO of a thriving fashion company with over 1,000 employees. I was married to a wonderful woman who supported me completely. We had a beautiful, healthy child, a home filled with warmth, and a future that seemed as bright as the Shanghai skyline. By all accounts, I was living the dream.

On the surface, I appeared to be thriving. But beneath the veneer of success, I was sinking deeper into physical and emotional exhaustion. The relentless pressure, endless hours, and unyielding stress of running a company with over 1,000 employees was taking a toll on my already sickly body. I could no longer ignore the signs.

At first, I convinced myself that this was the price of success—and I was willing to pay it. But as the years passed, my energy waned, and my health deteriorated. Eventually, the truth became undeniable: My career was destroying me.

After graduating from university, I had flaunted the traditional system and rejected the job that the government offered me at a state-run factory in order to pursue greater opportunities. For years, I struggled. Then I made a bold move: I signed an agreement with a foreign trading company to work on commission only, forgoing a salary in exchange for a 50-50 profit split. I assembled a team of three people, and we grew the business rapidly.

One of our most important clients was a prestigious Japanese wholesaler known for their exacting standards. They demanded higher quality products than our manufacturers were accustomed to producing. It became clear that if I wanted to continue growing the business, I would have to take control of the manufacturing process myself. So, in 1999, I founded my own apparel manufacturing company, starting with about 100 workers. With guidance from my Japanese client, the business thrived.

Two years later, we moved to a larger facility to accommodate our expanding operations. But as the business grew, so did the demands on my time and energy. Manufacturing requires long hours, and there were times when I had to work around the clock to meet shipping deadlines. I found myself managing customer orders, securing loans, and handling payroll, all while navigating complex relationships with the government. The strain was becoming unbearable.

One day, my wife, who has a medical degree, noticed something alarming. "Your face looks pale and has a slight yellowish tint, LD," she said. "You need to get tested."

The lab tests revealed that I had liver disease. The doctor prescribed medication, and I returned to work at once, determined to keep the business running.

It wasn't long before the company had expanded to 1,000 employees. Now I was responsible for paying 1,000 salaries every month, managing substantial debts, and facing increasing competition with razor-thin profit margins.

Soon, I began experiencing more disturbing symptoms. My heart would race unexpectedly, my chest felt constricted, and I could no longer move my neck freely. My back was in constant pain, and I was grappling with severe anxiety. The mere act of entering the factory filled me with dread.

I went to see the doctor again. The results of the tests were alarming: She told me that I was at serious risk of a dangerous, rare kind of heart attack—a condition that could strike without warning.

Around the same time, another specialist diagnosed me with asthma. The prognosis was grim. "We can prescribe medication," he said, "but recovery will be difficult."

The situation deteriorated even further. I could no longer drive for more than an hour without needing to lie down in the back seat. My neck was stiff, my back pain unbearable, and the daily pressure of running the business felt overwhelming.

It all came to a climax one evening when I collapsed in my bedroom, unable to breathe.

At the hospital the next day, I agreed with my wife: I had to do something, anything, to change the course of my life. Otherwise, it might end altogether.

In Beijing, I consulted with one of the best traditional Chinese medicine (TCM) doctors around, who was known for treating asthma. He prescribed a two-week course of herbs and acupuncture. Later, I returned to Beijing for another round. But despite following his treatment plan, nothing changed.

Fortunately, an opportunity presented itself. A passionate entrepreneur offered to buy me out of my manufacturing business. Although I continued to work under him, I no longer had to endure the long hours or relentless pressure of managing 1,000 employees.

With some of my stress alleviated, I focused further on my health. I joined a gym, started practicing Tai Chi, and diligently took nutritional supplements. But I still felt breathless and exhausted.

Then, one day, I noticed that my left leg was going numb. Concerned, I visited another doctor. She told me that while I could manage the condition, it could never be fully cured.

This news left me feeling truly desperate.

During my next Tai Chi session, I shared my struggles with my teacher. He listened carefully and then suggested something different: "Maybe you should try Oneness."

A New Beginning

"Oneness? *Really*?" I responded, eyebrows arching with skepticism. I had barely ever heard of it, much less known anyone who practiced it. Nevertheless, something within pushed me to explore further.

I turned to the Chinese equivalent of Amazon and purchased over 20 books on the subject of Oneness. After sifting through them, one book stood out: *Dacheng Chuanxilu*, authored by Grandmaster Yu Hongkun. Intrigued, I reached out to him. Following a month of correspondence, I traveled to Beijing to meet him in person.

When I first laid eyes on Mr. Yu, he seemed quite ordinary: Middle aged, tall and thin with a bit of a hunchback. But I was struck by his warmth and aura of serenity. At once, I felt close to him, as if meeting again an old friend I'd known since childhood. Even as I pestered him with question after question, he answered with clarity and patience. Gently, he trained me in the proper stance and encouraged me to simply give it a try. And so, I started practicing Oneness on a daily basis.

Oneness demands nothing more than standing still. Of course, there are a few more critical details. You relax your body, stand upright, and bring your awareness to the present moment. You smile slightly. As you grow more comfortable, you raise your arms a little. If you need more energy, you might add three short punches to your practice.

But it really is simple. Unbelievably simple.

Just don't mistake simple for weak or ineffective.

I Walk Through the Doorway

Unlike my father and grandfathers—all of whom were tall and strong—I was smaller and much weaker than I ought to have been. I frequently suffered from colds and fevers that required visits to doctors. Furthermore, I was born into the chaos of the Cultural Revolution. My family had been left in disarray, scattered, and I was raised by my maternal grandparents. They rarely allowed me to play outside with other children, so I spent most of my early years indoors and alone.

My body may have been stunted and my childhood may have been rife with trauma, yet in the end, I was loved. Looking back now, I can see how those difficulties actually planted seeds of resilience within me. My will was quietly growing stronger. It was this will that led me to seek treatment after treatment with conventional doctors and traditional Chinese medicine practitioners, refusing to take "no cure" for an answer. It was this will that guided me to Oneness. And it is this will that got me to a place of total healing of my mind, body and spirit.

Now, I watch my health and wellness blossom day after day. I am grateful for my strong will. Perhaps that is why I chose the American name "Will" Chen.

At first, I could only stand for five minutes. Gradually, I increased my endurance—first to 10 minutes, then 15, and eventually 30. Each time, my heels would ache slightly. Occasionally, I experienced discomfort in my joints and back. I would consult Grandmaster Yu for guidance.

"These are good signs," Grandmaster Yu told me. "The aches and slight discomfort indicate that energy is building up in your body and flowing through it, initiating the healing process."

With his support, I eventually reached the point where I could stand for an hour straight. As I did, I began feeling a deep sense of joy arising within me. What began as a task I felt I *had to* do transformed into something I looked forward to and enjoyed.

Over time, the discomforts I once had felt faded away. Along with them, so did numerous other health problems. I no longer experienced tightness in my chest from asthma or the irregular heartbeats that had plagued me. My neck, which used to stiffen painfully after sitting in a car, ceased bothering me.

The numbness in my leg disappeared as well. My anxiety dissipated significantly.

About six months after I began practicing Oneness, I went for a follow-up lab test. The results astonished my doctor: All traces of liver disease were gone from my body.

Not only that, but I became more resilient to illness in general, particularly colds and infections. In the past, my wife would joke that if someone in our circle caught a cold, I was guaranteed to catch it, too. But during the Covid pandemic, when every member of my family contracted the virus—some of them twice—I remained unaffected. Even when two of my son's classmates who were staying with us for the holidays fell ill with Covid, I did not.

I'm 55 this year, and I can honestly say that I wake up every day feeling happier, more at peace, and more energetic than I ever have before. This is why I am so excited to share the miracle of Oneness with you.

The Miracle of Oneness

I never expected this outcome.

When I was first introduced to Oneness, I questioned it. *How can standing still possibly cure my physical ailments? And if it really is just a practice of standing still, how is Oneness different from meditation?*

I will answer these and more questions later in the book. But for now, I will say this: After just a few weeks of practicing, I began asking myself a different question entirely: *How can a technique be so powerful, and yet so few people know about it?* I feel incredibly fortunate to have found my way to Oneness.

People accustomed to conventional medicine don't understand why Oneness works, so I explain it this way: Oneness is designed to heal you—body, mind and spirit. Every person is born with the innate wisdom and abilities to heal themselves, and Oneness practice is about awakening this inherent wisdom. It returns us to our natural state, cleansing us of all negative influences and allowing us to start anew with improved health, happiness, and more.

Imagine that your smartphone freezes. You can't access any of the apps or even make a call. You try everything to fix it, but nothing works. Then you switch it off and restart it. Suddenly, it works again.

Oneness reboots you. It brings you back to life.

Some people start to feel the changes right away, others within weeks of beginning to practice, others within months. But no matter what, if you keep up the practice, you will have more energy. Your mood improves. Your body begins to heal. You feel greater empathy toward others and have more love in your heart. This, in turn, impacts your relationships. You get along better with the people around you.

Over time, Oneness is totally life-changing. It transforms you into someone completely new. On the outside, you might still look the same—or just a little different. But inside, you're changed. You think differently. You react differently. You experience the world differently.

Through Oneness, it is possible to awaken, heal, and transform.

- If you're battling health conditions that modern medicine can't fix—I made it through, and so can you.
- If you rely on pills to survive—others have found lasting healing, and you can, too.
- If you're suffering from anxiety, burnout, or depression—many people have broken free, and so can you.
- If you're fighting chronic pain or arthritis—countless others have healed, and you can, too.
- If you want a clear mind and heightened awareness—many have experienced it, and so can you.

- If you desire more fulfilling, loving relationships—these are within your reach, too.
- If you're seeking awakening—you can go even further, surpassing what you previously imagined.
- If you're searching for a more joyful life—I've found it, and it's waiting for you.

All this is possible for you.

As you read on, you will learn more about my own life journey. You'll also discover numerous stories of people who have healed themselves through Oneness. I'll share scientific research and the ancient history of Oneness, and also highlight key differences between it and traditional Chinese medicine, martial arts, meditation, and biohacking.

Finally, I will explain how to stand, how to breathe, how to be present, and how to push past challenges in your practice. You will experience for yourself the power of non-doing, the magic of simply being.

If this book is in your hands right now, then I believe it must be for a reason. Read it. Try it. This book is not here to convince you of anything. This book is here to show you the doorway, so that you can experience the power of Oneness for yourself. It is up to you to step through it.

What have you got to lose? Unlock the power that already lives within you.

And if it works for you, please don't keep it to yourself. Share the book and the miracle of Oneness with someone you love—someone who is searching for hope.

PART I

The Power of Onenesss

Chapter 1

Muddy Water, Clear Sky

People are like muddy water.
Through the practice of Oneness,
the water becomes clear as the blue sky.
– Grandmaster Yu

Modern life is filled with noise, stress, and endless distractions. All too often, we find ourselves disconnected—from nature, from other people, from our bodies, and even from our own feelings. Meanwhile, we're driven to seek fulfillment through external achievements, experiencing intense societal pressure to get a higher paying job, buy a bigger house, and drive a fancier car.

As a result of this stress and strain, most people spend their lives reacting, pulled by their desires, fears, and the intense demands of just trying to get by. Unable to access inner peace, they numb themselves by drinking and taking prescription medications, gambling, shopping, and most of all, endlessly staring into their screens—playing video games, watching YouTube videos, and checking social media follower counts.

Small wonder mental health crises are on the rise, with anxiety, depression, and burnout reaching epidemic proportions in the past decade. Chronic illnesses such as diabetes, heart disease, and autoimmune disorders are becoming alarmingly commonplace. On a societal level, our relationships are fractured, our families are struggling, and our sense of purpose is eroding.

How many times have you found yourself apologizing after snapping at your partner or children, chalking it up to "having a bad day"? I've been there, too, regretting harsh words almost as soon as they left my lips. The true tragedy lies not in these individual moments, but in spending an entire lifetime weighed down by unhappiness and resentment, only to realize—when it's too late—that the ones you have hurt the most are those you love the most deeply.

You can find thousands of self-help books, alternative healers, therapists, conventional doctors, shamans, gurus, and retreat centers offering to guide you in fixing your life. And more than a few deliver helpful solutions.

But the fact of the matter is, most people simply don't have enough energy or free time to transform their lives through engaging in these practices. For someone already struggling from depression, pain, or chronic illness, it's nearly impossible to keep up with the demands of complicated programs and/or the long-term expense of pricey regimens.

Oneness offers a way out of this conundrum.

You stop searching for the right tools to cure your depression, help you overcome your illness, and change your life. You stop forcing yourself to figure out how to use them. Instead, you just let go. You relax into the joy of non-doing. And by simply being in stillness, at peace with yourself and the world, healing energy flows. Nature, mind and body unite.

A Simple Solution

What we have forgotten in today's world is that balance, clarity, and healing have been residing within us all along. Every single one of us can access a state life's struggles dissolve into peace. And Oneness offers a direct path to this state.

The key is energy.

Energy is the most important ingredient in helping you change your state, both mental and physical. And it is exactly what Oneness gives you. It activates your body's internal energy—the same life force refined by Kung Fu masters for centuries. This is energy you can harness to heal, recharge, and awaken your mind and body. And once your energy rises, everything in your life begins to change.

While it draws from ancient Chinese wisdom that has been cherished by Zen masters, Taoists, and Kung Fu practitioners for thousands of years, the wisdom of Oneness extends far beyond any single tradition. It is a one-stop shop. It strengthens your body. It clears your mind. It restores your spirit.

With Oneness practice, you find that your energy flows effortlessly. You begin to notice the tension in your shoulders dissolve—tension that you never even realized was there. You observe the way your breath flows, and note how it slows and deepens. You discover a silent strength hidden within the stillness.

As these changes unfold, something magical happens. Your body begins to heal itself. Vitality returns, and you discover an endless well of love and compassion that you quite possibly never knew existed within you. Your increased energy expands your awareness beyond your practice. You find that you can dissolve anger, halt arguments before they begin, and break free from the prison of judgment.

You shift from *reacting* to *being*. You become attuned to life itself.

"People are like muddy water," says my sensei, Grandmaster Yu. "Through the practice of Oneness, the water becomes clear as the blue sky."

Flowing through Life

When you engage fully in practicing Oneness with your body, you simultaneously train your mind and open your heart. The energy cultivated through Oneness naturally manifests outwardly, influencing how you think about and move through the world.

The beauty of this approach lies in its practicality. Unlike the advice in most self-help books, which demand that you *do this* or *stop that*—control your desires, let go of anger, follow endless rules—Oneness doesn't ask you to fight or fix anything. Like a Kung Fu master's effortless power during practice, you flow naturally through your life. Anger and desire lose their grip on you not because you suppress them, but because you become immune to them, untouched by their forcefulness. You don't have to manage your emotions, you just let them be.

The application of Oneness in your daily life is elegant in its simplicity. It doesn't require you to set aside hours for separate physical and mental training. Rather than adding yet another set of tasks to your already busy life, Oneness brings a different quality to what you are already doing. As you relax and allow yourself to feel the flow, every aspect of your life improves.

"When Oneness practice and life merge seamlessly, you discover that the clarity and strength cultivated in standing naturally inform how you engage with every aspect of your existence," Grandmaster Yu says. "You begin to see the essence of situations more clearly. You respond rather than react. You navigate challenges with a resilience that comes not from forcing outcomes, but from aligning with the natural flow of energy. And perhaps most meaningfully, you develop the capacity to help others find their way to this same state of integrated presence."

The true gift of Oneness is this ability to meet whatever arises with an open heart and clear mind. To stand firmly in your center even as life swirls around you. To find, as the ancient Taoist sages described it, stillness in movement and movement in stillness.

Oneness is such a deceptively straightforward practice. It requires no special equipment, no elaborate rituals. It does not involve biohacking or visits to numerous doctors or expensive supplements.

That said, please don't mistake the simplicity of Oneness for ease. The journey requires commitment and proper guidance as your body and mind undergo subtle yet profound transformations.

And, especially with proper guidance from a Oneness coach or sensei, you can embark on a continuous spiral of growth, reaching ever-greater heights of physical health, spiritual awakening, and inner peace. When this happens, you will find that you can move through life effortlessly.

Imagine standing on the edge of a vast ocean, watching as the water meets the horizon in perfect harmony. This is the essence of Oneness—a state of complete unity where the boundaries between body and mind, individual and universe, even between ourselves and those we consider to be our enemies dissolve. A state of selflessness.

The circular "O" at the start of the word "Oneness" serves as a powerful symbol of this wholeness, which blesses every person on earth. A regular practice enables you to transcend dualistic thinking and engage with the world without being disturbed by it, thus returning to this innate state of wholeness.

It seems like a miracle.

And it begins with just five minutes a day.

Chapter 2

Why Oneness Works

Healing doesn't have to be complicated.

Sarah had lived with the pain for so long that it had become like an old, unwelcome friend—always there, shifting its weight from one spot to another but never truly leaving. At 58, she had grown accustomed to planning her life around her monthly migraines, timing important work meetings and family gatherings around when she thought the pain might strike. Her medicine cabinet told a miserable story: Rows of painkillers and herbal remedies, each promising relief that never quite arrived.

Like many people who suffer from chronic conditions, Sarah had tried everything conventional medicine had to offer, as well as numerous solutions presented to her by doctors of Traditional Chinese Medicine (TCM). Yet the headaches that had plagued her since adolescence remained stubbornly present.

Then, on an otherwise ordinary Tuesday afternoon, Sarah discovered Oneness. A friend casually mentioned a local teacher offering free courses in the local park.

"It's just standing still?" Sarah asked skeptically. "How could that possibly help me?" But desperation has a way of opening doors we might otherwise pass by, so Sarah decided to give Oneness a try.

The first sessions were challenging. With no distractions, she felt every ache in her body cry out for attention. Her mind, untamed and restless, fought against the stillness. And so, her sensei suggested that Sarah add movement in order to get her energy flowing. He trained her in the Three Fists technique.

Sarah would stand still for a few breaths. Then, deliberately, she would take a step forward and punch the air with her right hand, left hand, right hand. After returning to a standing position, she would breathe and then repeat.

After just a few days, Sarah experienced a significant reduction in pain. "I slept like a baby for the first time in years!" she said. "I felt like I could take on my health challenges. Before, I just felt hopeless."

As weeks of Oneness practice turned into months, Sarah realized something extraordinary: Her migraines, those faithful tormentors for decades, had faded like footprints washing away on a beach.

Sarah's body, she realized, possessed innate wisdom. Given the right conditions, it could heal itself. Oneness provided these conditions, creating a space where energy could flow freely, where balance could be restored, and where her body could remember its natural state of wellness.

Although her healing didn't happen overnight, Sarah could not believe that simply by standing still and then punching the air three times with awareness, she had found her way to a pain-free life. Just a year ago, she never would have believed it possible.

The Evidence for Oneness

According to the National Institutes of Health (NIH), there are somewhere between 7,000 and 10,000 diseases affecting humans, of which only about 500 have any U.S. Food and Drug Administration-approved treatment.

The conventional medical system excels at treating acute diagnostic issues such as high cholesterol or a broken bone. But more often than not, it fails to cure more nebulous issues such as chronic health conditions and mental illnesses. This is where Oneness comes into play.

Preliminary research suggests that a regular Oneness practice may be able to:

- **Boost brain function**: Increase blood flow to the brain, particularly in areas associated with attention, memory, and emotional regulation. This may contribute to improved cognitive function.
- **Improve cardiovascular health**: Lower blood pressure, improve circulation, reduce heart rate variability, and improve heart rate recovery after exercise. These effects may contribute to a reduced risk of cardiovascular disease.
- **Reduce stress and anxiety**: Decrease levels of the stress hormone cortisol, and increase levels of endorphins, which serves to reduce anxiety and depression and leads to better sleep.
- **Lead to better balance and posture**: Enhance balance, coordination, and posture, which is particularly beneficial for older adults and individuals with balance impairments.
- **Improve digestion**: Simulate the functioning of the digestive system.
- **Increase energy levels**: Heighten energy and reduce fatigue. This may be due to several factors noted above, including improved circulation, reduced stress, and enhanced energy flow.
- **Reduce inflammation**: Alleviate chronic inflammation by promoting balanced circulation and enhanced immune responses. This helps reduce symptoms such as pain, swelling, and fatigue.

- **Boost metabolism**: Enhance cellular activity and immune system response. Regular practitioners sometimes exhibit increased red and white blood cell counts and improved circulation.
- **Calm the nervous system:** EEG studies show that Oneness can reduce overactive brain signals, leading to deeper relaxation, improved self-regulation, less anxiety and better sleep.

Unfortunately, unlike modern medicine with its surgeries, pills and vaccines, scientific research into Oneness is more challenging. It harnesses energy flow for healing, addressing the interconnectedness of body, mind, and spirit in a way that science is only beginning to understand. Researchers have not yet determined a methodology for measuring energy flow. Furthermore, every individual is different, meaning that the body's response to Oneness can vary significantly between people, even for the same condition.

That said, scientific studies conducted by Chinese medical institutions including Beijing University, China's most respected research institution, as well as the Beijing Railway Affiliated Hospital, Beijing Iron and Steel Hospital, and the Chinese Medicine Research Institute in Hebei Province reveal that Oneness has been successfully applied to treat a wide range of disorders.

At the First Affiliated Hospital of Beijing Medical University, a comprehensive study was conducted on 18 people. After incorporating Oneness into their treatments, 84% of participants experienced significant improvements to their health, including reduced symptoms of dizziness and headaches, a sense of overall physical relaxation, better sleep quality, increased appetite, and enhanced emotional well-being.

Typically, people begin to experience these benefits after just days or weeks of consistent practice. Some may also experience muscle soreness, trembling, numbness, swelling, belching, stomach rumbling, and other phenomena. These are normal reactions, indicating that your body is undergoing repair. They will gradually dissipate over time, replaced by a delightful state of effortless flow.

I cannot promise that you will experience such results. Please do not consider this book a substitute for professional medical advice. You should always consult a doctor when beginning any new regimen. That said, I have watched many people recover from chronic illness and severe mental health challenges through Oneness. It really is incredible.

Change your Body, Change your Mind

Changing your mind takes a lot of energy. Most people who are stuck, depressed, anxious, or suffering from pain and illness can't do it through sheer willpower.

So, change your physiology first. Change the way you move, breathe, and stand.

Here's an example researched by Harvard Business School professor Amy Cuddy. Her research has revealed that adopting a "power pose"—throwing your shoulders back and holding your head high for as little as two minutes—can help you feel more powerful and less stressed. Your testosterone levels increase by 20% in two minutes, which helps you focus, enhances your memory, and contributes to you being 33% more likely to take action.

This is similar to how Oneness works. You start with your posture. From posture, energy flows. From energy flow, healing happens.

It is just that simple.

Why Complicate Healing?

Healing doesn't have to be complicated.

By harmonizing the body's energy, Oneness allows us to cure ourselves from the inside, addressing the root causes of our health issues rather than just the symptoms.

Not only that, but Oneness nurtures a deep connection between mind and body. Your thoughts slow down, your body releases tension. This fosters a tranquility that carries over into your daily life, leading to greater clarity, peace, and fulfillment.

Best of all, unlike other practices focused on gaining strength and flexibility or mastering complex movements, Oneness is accessible to everyone, regardless of age, physical condition, and experience level. Whether you're seeking healing, mental clarity, or spiritual growth, Oneness meets you where you are. You don't even need to be able to stand—you can practice Oneness lying down if need be.

Many people continue to practice long after they have achieved the physical and mental healing that initially brought them to Oneness. They experience profound transformation, letting go of old wounds, improving their relationships, and experiencing nothing short of a spiritual awakening.

This is the power of Oneness. It reveals the deeper potential that resides within all of us.

Chapter 3

Who Oneness Is For

Oneness is one for all.

When Jason, a 42-year-old tech entrepreneur, received his diagnosis, the gravity of his situation hit him like a physical blow. His blood pressure had reached dangerously high levels—so high that all three specialists he consulted delivered the same verdict: He needed immediate bypass surgery.

"It felt like my body was betraying me just at the moment when my business was finally taking off," Jason recalls. "The doctors made it clear surgery wasn't optional. Without intervention, I was looking at a stroke or heart attack, possibly within months."

But for the next few days, Jason researched alternatives during sleepless nights. That's when he discovered Oneness. "It seemed too simple to be effective," he admits. "Just standing still? But I was desperate enough to try anything that might help me avoid surgery."

With nothing to lose, Jason sought out a training program and began practicing Oneness daily, standing in the basic posture for 20 minutes each morning and evening. The first week was challenging—his legs trembled, his feet ached, and his mind raced with doubts. But by the second week, something began to shift.

"I noticed I was breathing more deeply throughout the day. Not only that, but I felt the stress of my work ease. I was relaxed yet energized," he says.

After just three weeks of consistent practice, Jason returned to his doctor for a follow-up appointment. Both he and his physician were stunned by the results: His blood pressure had dropped so significantly that surgery was no longer considered necessary.

"My doctor couldn't explain it," Jason says, shaking his head. "He asked what medication I was taking, and when I told him none—just Oneness practice—he thought I was joking."

Two years later, Jason continues his daily practice. His blood pressure remains stable without medication, and he's become an advocate for Oneness among his high-stress colleagues in the tech industry.

"What began as a desperate alternative to surgery has become the foundation of my well-being," he reflects. "Sometimes the simplest solutions really are the most powerful."

When All Else Fails

Jason's story is not an isolated incident. His results can be attributed to a practice that has been quietly honed and perfected for thousands of years—a practice that is available to you now for the first time.

Over and over again, students of Oneness say the same thing: They've tried medication. They've tried surgery, acupuncture, chiropractic treatments, vitamins and supplements. They've tried other practices, like meditation, yoga and Tai Chi.

Sometimes they get temporary relief. But because they don't have enough energy, none of these tactics results in permanent change.

Then they start practicing Oneness, and they feel something different. They experience real, lasting change—even though the practice is so much simpler than the other techniques they have tried.

"I can't believe it," remarked a woman in her 50s with severe diabetes. She had already lost one leg, and the toes on her remaining leg had gone completely numb. Thanks to Oneness, sensation returned to her toes and her diabetes slowly disappeared.

"It's magic," exclaimed a young student who had suffered from crippling back pain for over a decade. She couldn't bend at the waist. After practicing Oneness for just a few months, her pain evaporated. She could touch her toes.

Each person's story ignites my soul because I have felt the same joy—I've been where these individuals have been, and I've benefited from Oneness in the same way. Hearing about their experiences fuels my calling. I know there are millions more people out there who are desperate for a solution, just like they were.

People like you.

Oneness is for People Seeking Healing

Like Jason and myself, many people initially come to Oneness seeking healing. These are individuals suffering from physical ailments, mental illness, or both. In almost every case, modern medicine has failed them. Their persistent pain, autoimmune disorders, diabetes, depression and suicidal ideation, debilitating anxiety, and other conditions have defied conventional treatments.

According to numerous testimonials and a growing body of medical research, Oneness practice has been shown to have a potential significant impact on a variety of conditions, including:

- Insomnia
- Heart disease

- High blood pressure
- Diabetes
- Anxiety
- Depression
- Respiratory issues
- Digestive problems
- Gastroenteritis
- Neurasthenia
- Arthritis
- Liver disease
- Chronic pain
- Climacteric syndrome
- Thyroid issues
- Cancer recovery
- Post-chemo care to prevent metastasis
- And other rare and unnamed conditions

Oneness is for People Seeking Performance Enhancement

Another category of people who train in Oneness are those seeking to enhance their performance. Traditional Chinese Medicine (TCM) doctors may use Oneness to heal themselves and to sharpen their diagnostic skills. The practice heightens their ability to sense subtle changes in the body's energy, enabling accurate diagnoses without relying on expensive lab tests and X-rays.

A renowned *guqin* player is a disciple of Mr. Yu. Musicians, artists, and other creative professionals use Oneness to clear their minds to better accomplish their work. The practice deepens their connection with their instruments, their music, and their audience, thereby enhancing their output, performances and enjoyment.

All kinds of athletes, from golfers to baseball players, and their coaches use Oneness to optimize their full physical potential. The practice helps them achieve better focus, balance, and internal strength, giving them a competitive edge.

Oneness also serves as the foundation for martial arts practitioners who are interested in building their internal power, stamina, and mental clarity. These students are often already skilled in other martial arts but seek the deeper, more subtle power that Oneness offers. They understand that true mastery comes from within, and Oneness is the path to cultivating that inner strength.

Oneness is for People Seeking Spiritual Growth and Wellbeing

Another sizable group of students are on a quest for spiritual growth, awakening, or enlightenment. For them, Oneness practice offers a way to connect deeply with God, the Universe, or the Tao, to reduce the sense of self, and to harmonize with the natural flow of life. Through dedicated practice, they aspire to achieve a state of non-doing (*wu wei*), where actions arise naturally and effortlessly from a place of inner stillness and awareness.

Lastly, some students do not begin with a specific ailment or goal, but rather feel a general sense of unease or dissatisfaction with life. Drawn to Oneness for its calming and centering effects, they find that engaging in the practice is like using a boat to cross a river: It serves as a vehicle to take you to the other bank—a place of greater balance, peace, and joy.

Fundamentally, they are all seeking transformation.

Oneness is for all. Your body and your mind become one. You and nature, the world around you, become one. You and other people become one. You, as a human being, and the universe become one.

PART II

The History of
Oneness

Chapter 4

Taoist Origins

Stop fighting with life, and begin dancing with it instead.

Since long ago in China, Oneness has been cultivated by Taoist, Zen and Kung Fu masters, transcending any specific philosophy. Although it is an ancient practice, Oneness is not a religion, nor is it tied to any specific philosophy. Rather, it is a universal methodology accessible to anyone, regardless of age, physical mobility, mental health challenges, race, religion, economic status or family background. It offers a portal to a parallel universe—one where pain, anxiety, and suffering are replaced by peace, contentment, and a deep connection to the world around you.

Let's journey into the past to understand the origins of Oneness, and the quest to unlock the hidden potential that lies within every human soul.

We begin with Taoism.

When we are born, the Taoists believe, we exist in a harmonious state, fully integrated with nature. Think of how babies giggle in glee, scream in purple-faced protest, and poop in their diapers without the slightest hint of hesitation or embarrassment. As we grow older, however, our minds and bodies warp under the continuous influence of parental expectations, societal concepts, and other environmental factors.

This is particularly true in modern times, when we have become far removed from the source of life due to spending most of our time indoors and on screens. As we age, if we do not make appropriate adjustments, our mind and body drift further and further away from our original, natural state. This disconnection manifests physically as stiffness, chronic illness, infertility, and diseases such as cancer. Mentally it manifests as stress, anxiety, depression, addiction, and other challenges.

The ancient Chinese philosophy of Taoism teaches us to seek out a harmonious balance between body, mind, and the energy of life. It encourages us to return to our original, natural state of being.

Oneness is a way to do just that.

The Tao Te Ching

Taoism emerged during what historians call the Axial Age (8th century BCE to 1st century CE), a remarkable period when humanity experienced simultaneous spiritual awakenings across different civilizations and continents: The Buddha attained enlightenment in India; Jesus Christ preached compassion for all people in the Middle East; and in China, Confucius taught about the importance of social order and proper relationships.

Also around the 3rd or 4th century BCE in China, the sage Lao Tzu wrote the *Tao Te Ching* (*The Book of The Way*), a poetic text that continues to inspire millions of people worldwide with its elegant simplicity. Within its verses, we discover the essence of what would eventually evolve into Oneness practice—living in harmony with the natural order of the universe without resisting.

The key to Taosim is "going with the flow," as Westerners are fond of saying. What does this mean?

Imagine yourself swimming in a great river. When you struggle against the current, you exhaust yourself. But if you surrender and allow the river to carry you, all the while maintaining your awareness and gently floating on the surface of the water, you will discover a way of moving through life with grace and power.

This represents the Taoist principle of *wu wei* or *non-doing*. It is not a state of passive resignation, but rather one of aligned action wherein your results emerge effortlessly because you trust in nature's intelligence to take you exactly where you need to be.

The principle of non-doing and flowing with the energy of life can be further conveyed by the following Chinese parable.

The Farmer's Folly

Once, in a small village, there lived a rice farmer. He planted the seeds in his field and impatiently awaited a bountiful harvest. Every morning, he ventured out into the watery rice paddies to check on the plants' progress. But as the days passed, no green shoots emerged.

Frustrated by this situation, the farmer decided to take matters into his own hands. He walked into the field and tugged at each tiny sprout in order to make them taller. By the end of the day, he stood at the edge of his field, admiring his efforts.

"Look how much taller the plants are now!" he told his son. "I am a genius. I have made the rice grow faster."

The next morning, the farmer's son rushed to the field to see how much taller the rice had grown. Instead, he found that all the rice plants had withered and died. The farmer wept in despair. His intervention had disrupted the natural growth cycle of the rice plants, whose delicate roots could no longer sustain them.

The moral of this story is that nature follows its own rhythm, and we must trust in that in our everyday lives. Trying to force outcomes only leads to destruction.

Taoist Principles of Oneness

Taoism has always been intimately connected to physical health as well as spiritual growth and awakening. The practices that evolved from it, including Oneness, offer a tangible way to reduce the dominance of the ego and harmonize with life's natural rhythms.

What makes Oneness so effective is how it integrates Taoist wisdom with structured methods accessible to modern practitioners. By encouraging us to let go of forcing and striving, it creates space for the body and mind to heal naturally. Each session becomes an opportunity to reconnect with our original, harmonious state of being—the state of integration with nature that we were born into, before tension and conditioning began to separate us from the Tao.

Oneness cultivates what Taoists call *inner power*—a quality of presence and vitality that emanates from within, rather than being imposed from without. True to Taoist principles, this power isn't developed for dominance. On the contrary, the aim is for us to live in harmony with ourselves and others. It's the same energy that allows a blade of grass to push through concrete or a tree to gradually split a boulder—not through force but through consistent, aligned presence.

I've witnessed this principle transform the lives of many people in Oneness workshops. One participant, a corporate executive named Sam who approached everything as a battle to be won, discovered that his chronic health issues, including high blood pressure and heart disease, stemmed from this resistance. As he learned to practice Oneness, his body gradually released decades of accumulated tension.

"I'm doing less, but I'm accomplishing more," Sam told me with wonder in his eyes. "All the while, I feel peaceful inside."

The concept of *yang sheng* (nurturing life) represents another profound Taoist contribution to Oneness. In ancient China, a culture of health wasn't reserved for rulers and specialists, but was considered important for everyone. The *Tao Te Ching* emphasizes that cultivating good physical health forms an essential part of the spiritual path. It serves as a foundation for deeper awakening.

Oneness practice connects body and mind. The standing posture of Oneness aligns closely with the body's natural physiological structure, allowing the internal organs to relax in their normal positions, the bones and joints to fall comfortably in place, and the body's energy channels (known in TCM as *meridians*) to flow smoothly.

Perhaps the most challenging aspect of Taoist practice involves letting go of the self. "Empty your mind of all thoughts, let your heart be at peace," advises the *Tao Te Ching*.

Beyond the poetic language, this serves as a practical instruction. The greatest obstacle to our well-being is often our own ego. Its biases, fears, and attachments constrain our physical bodies and decimate our minds, leading to disease and unhappiness.

I've struggled with this aspect of Taoist teaching myself. As someone who built a career on knowledge and achievement, releasing my grip on the ego felt terrifying at first. Yet through consistent Oneness practice, I began to dissolve the boundaries between myself and the world around me, revealing a spaciousness where healing could naturally occur. This has proven to be the most profound medicine.

The beauty of the Taoist foundation of Oneness is that it requires no belief system or dogma. It simply invites us to notice what happens when we stop fighting against life and begin dancing with it instead.

Chapter 5

An Ancient Secret Revealed

In the past, people understood the principle of balance.

Huangdi, the Yellow Emperor, ruled China more than 4,000 years ago and remains one of its most celebrated rulers to this day. A renowned book about his teachings published 2,000 years ago called *Huangdi Neijing,* or *The Yellow Emperor's Inner Classic,* serves as the foundational text of Traditional Chinese Medicine.

The book tells this story.

One day, Huangdi said to his teacher Qi Bo, "I've heard the ancient peoples lived to be over one hundred years old without showing any signs of aging. In our time, people only live 50 years. Is this due to changes in the environment?"

"In the past, people understood the principle of balance," Qi Bo replied. "You must integrate the body, mind and spirit as one."

Oneness is a powerful way to do just that.

Why the Secrecy?

Despite the profound impact of Oneness on mind and body, for many centuries it remained a closely guarded secret among Taoist, Kung Fu, and Zen masters. It was transmitted only to a handful of dedicated disciples who demonstrated readiness for powerful inner transformation.

Why was this the case?

Perhaps it is because these spiritual traditions emphasize quiet cultivation and inner transformation—journeys that are by nature deeply personal, not commonly shared, and certainly not easily commercialized. Furthermore, the Oneness teachings were reserved only for those who demonstrated exceptional dedication and discipline.

As a result, knowledge of Oneness was kept to small, insular communities that followed specific lineages, passed down from generation to generation of sensei to student without written documentation. The practice remained largely inaccessible to the public.

That all changed in the mid-20th century thanks to Grandmaster Wang Xiangzhai, the founder of a Chinese martial art called *Dacheng Quan*.

From Sickly Child to Martial Arts Master

Born in 1886, Wang Xiangzhai was a sickly child. His parents, desperate to improve his health, sent him to train under Grandmaster Guo Yunshen, a renowned Chinese martial arts instructor.

When he arrived, Wang was eager to learn martial arts. Instead, Guo instructed the boy in *Zhan Zhuang*, the ancient standing still practice that serves as the foundation of what would later come to be known as *Dacheng Quan* and Oneness. The results were nothing short of remarkable. Wang regained his health completely. Grandmaster Guo then began training the boy in martial arts, as well.

Later, Wang Xiangzhai set off to travel across China. He wanted to study numerous martial arts disciplines from as many of the grandmasters as possible—Shaolin, Tai Chi, Bagua, and more. By the early 20th century, he had earned recognition as one of the greatest martial arts masters in Asia.

And yet Wang Xiangzhai was not satisfied. Returning to the essence of Zhan Zhuang, he eliminated all unnecessary movement from multiple martial arts disciplines, creating a new form based on the ancient standing still practice. This was named by his fellow martial arts masters as Dacheng Quan, meaning The Great Achievement Martial Art.

In the 1950s, Grandmaster Wang Xiangzhai began teaching Dacheng Quan and Zhan Zhuang across China. People sought training in Zhan Zhuang when neither conventional nor Traditional Chinese medicine could help cure their illnesses. It spread rapidly.

Some of Wang Xiangzhai's disciples even began incorporating Zhan Zhuang into their treatments in Chinese hospitals. According to my sensei's records, it proved to be more than 90% effective in healing almost any complaint.

Wang Xiangzhai had started a movement.

Chapter 6

The Next Generations

Let go of doing entirely and just be.

As Zhan Zhuang gained popularity across China, the second generation of practitioners emerged, including several notable people. The most famous of Grandmaster Wang Xiangzhai's disciples, the one who did the most to share the ancient practice with the world, was Grandmaster Wang Xuanjie.

From Debilitating Illness to Oneness Evangelist

Not unlike Grandmaster Wang Xiangzhai, who was sick for much of his childhood, Wang Xuanjie also suffered from poor physical health when he was young. A debilitating illness had left him so weak that he was unable to perform even the simplest tasks. Desperate for a cure, he turned to martial arts, studying under several renowned masters.

But it was not until the mid-1940s, when he became a disciple of Grandmaster Wang Xiangzhai and discovered the practice of Dacheng Quan, that Wang Xuanjie experienced a profound transformation. His body healed. Not only that, but he developed extraordinary martial arts prowess.

Over time, Grandmaster Wang Xuanjie defeated numerous challengers. He also trained many patients suffering from severe chronic diseases in Zhan Zhuang, thereby helping them to heal. Throughout his lifetime, he authored ten books on the subject, furthering the influence and legacy of a once-secret ancient practice.

My Sensei

My sensei, Grandmaster Yu Hongkun, represents the third generation of Dacheng Quan. I feel very fortunate to be his disciple.

In his younger days, Yu Hongkun was a martial arts champion in Sanda, a form of Chinese mixed martial arts (MMA) that involves boxing, kickboxing and wrestling. He loved it so much that he even pursued a master's degree in Chinese martial arts, studying Tai Chi and Buddhism, Taoism and traditional Chinese culture along the way.

Nevertheless, Yu wanted to discover an even more powerful martial art, one that would allow him to defeat opponents much larger in size. He set out on a quest. This is when he encountered Dacheng Quan and became a disciple of Grandmaster Wang Xuanjie.

Yu loved Dacheng Quan—especially the foundational practice of Zhan Zhuang, or standing still. He found that in Sanda and other martial arts, it was difficult for him to let go of his ego attachment to winning. He always wanted to defeat more opponents and attain more accolades. The true essence of Zhan Zhuang was to let go of any desire, to let go of doing entirely and just be.

As he dove deeper into Zhan Zhuang, Yu discovered that as this formerly secretive practice had spread to more people over the past few decades, it had grown increasingly complex and diluted. Many teachers did not stay true to the core principle of non-doing. Returning to the original form—the form he saw as the true lineage of the ancient practice—he renamed it *Li Chan Zhan Zhuang*. I translate this into English as *Oneness*.

Grandmaster Yu believes that true Oneness is boundless, a practice without direction that is infinitely adaptable. Applied to Kung Fu, it can unleash extraordinary power. Used for healing, it is profoundly transformative. In terms of spiritual awakening, it is unsurpassed.

In the past few decades, Grandmaster Yu has authored seven books on Oneness, which are popular in China today. He has also developed a training system and offers in-person retreats across the country. He has helped tens of thousands of people lead healthier, happier lives.

A Global Movement

Over the past two decades, global interest in alternative and holistic health practices has exploded. As people become increasingly disillusioned with the limitations of conventional medicine in addressing chronic conditions, they are turning to alternative approaches that offer a more integrative and holistic perspective on health.

Among these, according to numerous patient testimonials, Oneness stands out for its effectiveness not only in healing physical ailments and mental health issues, but also for leading to spiritual awakening.

The rise of global communication and the internet has further facilitated the sharing of this once-secret knowledge. Today, Oneness is practiced by people all over China, and its benefits are recognized by a growing number of scientists, doctors, and practitioners.

Now, it is time to bring Oneness to the West.

PART III

The Mechanisms
of Oneness

Chapter 7

Holistic: Oneness & Conventional Medicine

Over 90% of Oneness practitioners report significant improvements to their health without any side effects.

When Lin walked into her doctor's office in 2019, her prognosis was grim. She had fallen victim to diabetes, as had members of her family for generations. At age 54, she had already lost one leg and two fingers to amputation due to the disease. Now, Lin faced the unthinkable prospect of losing her other leg, as well. Not only that, but the three remaining fingers on her left hand were rapidly losing sensation—a telltale sign that her doctor would have to remove them soon.

The situation was even more dire due to a cruel twist of fate: Lin was allergic to anesthesia. Her doctor would not be able to put her fully under during the surgical procedure. The thought of remaining partially conscious during a second amputation, hearing the surgical tools at work and smelling the blood, filled Lin with profound dread.

It was this moment of crisis that pushed her to explore alternative paths to healing. In her search for solutions, Lin discovered Oneness. She traveled to Kunming, the capital city of Yunnan province in the southwest of China, to train with Grandmaster Yu. Though Oneness is traditionally performed standing up, Mr. Yu adapted the practice to accommodate Lin's physical limitations, guiding her to practice in a seated position.

Immediately, Lin felt a deep connection between mind, body, and the universal life force that flows through all things. She began a daily ritual of Oneness, which rapidly transformed into something extraordinary. After only a few months of consistent practice, she noticed subtle changes in the three fingers of her left hand and her toes. The numbness that had been creeping through them began to recede, replaced by vibrant sensation.

During her next medical evaluation, Lin's doctor was stunned by her reports of improved circulation and sensitivity in her extremities. He ran a series of tests, which showed measurable improvements in areas where deterioration had previously seemed inevitable. Contrary to all conventional medical expectations, her condition had stabilized. There was no longer any need for amputation.

Today, Lin continues her daily Oneness practice. Her diabetes has become less and less of a burden on her life. Her story has inspired her doctor to recommend Oneness to many other patients coping with diabetes.

The Limits of Conventional Medicine

During the past 70 years, the majority of practitioners turned to Oneness because they suffered from chronic health conditions that modern medicine could not effectively treat, from diabetes to depression, back pain to insomnia. According to reports from Chinese sources, over 90% of them report significant improvements without any side effects. Although detailed records—such as the exact duration and frequency of their practice—are scarce due to the wide variety of health conditions and lack of systematic tracking, these results speak for themselves. For many people, Oneness works.

The question is, why does something so simple lead to healing, where advanced conventional medicine often fails? That is the question we explore in this chapter.

Let me be clear: Conventional medicine is a miracle. Modern medical doctors can help infertile couples have babies, cure cancer, perform stem cell transplants, repair broken bones, conduct organ transplants and open-heart surgery, and develop vaccines to protect us from terrible diseases.

But when it comes to chronic pain and mysterious illnesses like Lyme disease and long Covid, as well as mental health challenges such as depression and anxiety, modern medicine frequently falls flat.

Perhaps a fundamental flaw is the approach to the human body. Conventional medicine focuses on closed systems and linear relationships. It treats the body as a complex machine, where each part can be pulled apart, studied, treated, and repaired independently, often by isolating and targeting specific symptoms.

Human biology, however, is an open and complex system. Attempting to understand it in purely mechanistic terms is an exercise doomed to failure, and often leads to one of two outcomes: If the disease has a simple, single cause and the treatment is minimal, the body recovers. But if the disease is complex and the symptoms don't provide clear guidance, the treatment becomes a gamble. It might help the patient but need to be performed for life, or it might not work at all. Worst case scenario, it upsets the body's delicate balance and deteriorates the patient's health.

Furthermore, many people experience discomfort without clear symptoms, and even advanced diagnostic tools like lab tests and X-rays fail to identify the cause. In such cases, modern medicine is extremely limited, capable of treating only the symptoms.

This is why conventional doctors usually struggle to treat chronic diseases caused by environmental, social, and psychological factors, or even genetics.

A Different Paradigm

Oneness offers a different paradigm. It works in harmony with the body's natural energy system to promote self-healing.

Key differences between Oneness and conventional medicine include:

1. **Acting on root causes vs. symptoms**: Whereas modern medicine targets treating symptoms through medication or surgery, Oneness focuses on restoring balance to the body's energy systems. Practitioners of Oneness discover how to completely surrender the Self, allowing energy to flow. This help heal the root cause of the problem.

2. **Treating the whole system vs. isolated parts**: Modern medicine usually isolates ailments and breaks the body into separate parts, whereas Oneness promotes the well-being of the entire bodily system by improving energy flow.

3. **Enhancing the body's own healing mechanisms vs. relying on external factors**: With modern medicine, recovery depends on surgery and medication. But Oneness strengthens the body's defenses from the inside out, enabling the body to heal itself.

Note: Please do not consider this chapter to be medical advice. I am in no way suggesting that you avoid or stop treatment by a conventional doctor. Oneness does not supplant traditional medicine, but can be practiced in conjunction with it.

Chapter 8

Harmonious:
Oneness & Traditional Chinese Medicine

Society has become like muddy water—lacking self-awareness.

In contrast to conventional medicine, which chases symptoms and treats isolated parts of the body, Traditional Chinese Medicine (TCM) views the body as a holistic entity. It respects the body's innate healing potential, making adjustments to restore balance and strengthen its energy, and thereby enabling you to overcome disease naturally.

Central to Taoism is the concept of *wu wei,* or non-doing. *Wu wei* is not about passivity, but rather aligning yourself with the natural flow of the universe, achieving results effortlessly by allowing actions to emerge harmoniously. This philosophy is deeply embedded in TCM. It is also a core principle of Oneness. Oneness also works on an energetic level.

Why, then, does TCM sometimes prove ineffective in healing people from chronic disorders?

The Modernization of a Traditional Practice

Unfortunately, in China today, TCM has been largely supplanted by modern medicine. In the beginning, TCM did not rely on lab tests, X-rays, or specialized departments. But in a world that has become like muddy water—lacking self-awareness—even doctors of traditional Chinese medicine are forced to rely heavily on these diagnostic tools.

As a result, when TCM is taught in universities in China, teachers now begin with anatomy and biology rather than classic texts like the *Huangdi Neijing* and the *Tao Te Ching*, which emphasize understanding and respecting the body's natural harmony.

This shift is why I was disappointed when one of the most renowned TCM doctors for asthma in all of China failed to treat my health issues—asthma, liver disease, and leg numbness. It wasn't until I read a book by a student of Dr. Li Ke that I understood fully what was happening.

Dr. Li was one of the most respected TCM doctors of the last 50 years. Wrongly imprisoned at age 23 and only released at 50, he spent those years studying all the major classic traditional Chinese medicine texts. Upon his release, he launched a practice, curing tens of thousands of patients who had been declared "incurable" by major hospitals. His approach was simple: Use Chinese herbal medicine to boost the patient's energy, then allow the body's own strength to overcome the disease.

Dr. Li's work convinced me that even in a modern world dominated by technology, the ancient wisdom of the Tao, with its emphasis on non-doing, still holds true. While most major Chinese hospitals have adopted modern practices, there are still a few practitioners who adhere to the original principles of TCM because it works. The problem is, it can be challenging to find those doctors of TCM who are firmly rooted in the ancient ways.

Meanwhile, there is Oneness.

Chapter 9

Effortless: Oneness & Martial Arts

Embrace a new definition of strength—
one that doesn't always display itself in visible ways.

"I once had a pet German Shepherd, a very strong dog," Grandmaster Yu said to his students. "One day, I was taking her for a walk by the beach as usual. Suddenly, a gust of wind blew, and the dog froze. She lay down on the ground, refusing to move."

"Confused, I looked around for what could have made my courageous dog cower like this," Yu continued. "Then ahead of us, I saw an old, frail tiger that had been retired from a circus. It was being used for photo sessions with tourists. Having smelled this tiger, my dog was terrified."

"Now tell me, did the tiger need training in any technique to intimidate my dog?" Yu inquired. "Did the tiger know any special moves?"

We students shook our heads no.

"Of course not!" Yu chuckled. "The tiger has innate power. Its power is a natural, effortless emanation of its true nature."

"And what does this have to do with Oneness?" one student asked.

"This story illuminates the difference between Oneness and martial arts," replied Grandmaster Yu. "Oneness is not about acquiring external techniques. It is about uncovering the internal power that already exists within us."

The Zero Point

Most of us are fascinated by the showy aspects of martial arts—the flying kicks, the lightning-fast punches, the elaborate forms that showcase a person's physical prowess and technical skill. We admire the disciplined bodies of the practitioners, their flexibility, strength, and coordination. These elements are undeniably impressive and valuable in their own right.

Instruction in traditional martial arts typically begins with these techniques—specific movements, forms, and applications that students must learn, practice, and refine for years. This approach is tangible and measurable, which appeals to the modern mindset. You can see yourself improving as you master more complex movements. There's a clear sense of progression, of adding to your repertoire.

Oneness takes the opposite approach. Rather than adding, it subtracts. Rather than learning new movements, you unlearn habitual patterns. The aim is to return to what Grandmaster Yu calls "the zero-point baseline"—a foundational state of pure awareness without preconceived notions.

I struggled with this concept for months when I first began practicing Oneness. As a high achiever who was always striving to be the best in school and my career, the idea of stripping everything away felt counterintuitive, threatening even. What would be left? Who would I be without my hard-earned accomplishments?

But after about five days of studying Oneness with Grandmaster Yu, I began to understand how there was no strategy and very little technique to it. Unlike martial arts, Oneness was not about mastering yet another skillset. Instead, a seamless flow state seemed to arise from nowhere and everywhere all at once.

"You've found it," Grandmaster Yu said. "The zero point."

Taoists call it *wu wei*—the principle of non-doing. It's the understanding that the most profound power comes not from forceful action, but from aligning with the natural flow of life's energy. Oneness creates the conditions for this alignment to occur, allowing energy to generate naturally without imposition or control.

Mind-Body Integration

This zero-point aspect of Oneness can prove deeply challenging for newcomers with backgrounds in the more dynamic martial arts. Initially, they may dismiss the practice as boring and pointless.

But Oneness has its advantages.

Martial arts tend to separate physical training from mental discipline. You learn techniques with your body, then separately cultivate mental focus, strategic thinking, and emotional control. Even when these elements are taught together, they often remain conceptually distinct—physical training for the body, meditation for the mind.

Similarly, many other spiritual or meditation practices focus exclusively on the mind, paying little attention to the body, which is viewed solely as a stable base for awareness. The result can be a fragmented approach whereby either the body becomes strong while the mind remains vulnerable, or the mind develops clarity while the body lacks vitality.

Oneness offers a radically integrated alternative. You don't train the body and mind separately, but rather you awaken the mind through the body. The physical posture serves as a gateway to energy cultivation, which in turn facilitates the mind's natural release of attachment, tension, and limitation.

This integration explains why Oneness can feel so direct and immediate, especially when compared to martial arts. It doesn't require you to master any moves first. It addresses the whole person from the very beginning.

Accessibility

Finally, the fact that Oneness does not require you to perform any fancy postures, elaborate movements, or special techniques means that it is accessible. Anyone can practice Oneness, regardless of physical disability or mental health constraint. It doesn't even have to be performed standing up! It can be done seated or lying on the ground, if necessary.

If you're coming to Oneness from a background in martial arts—whether it's Kung Fu, Karate, Tai Chi, or any other discipline—I invite you to approach this practice with an open mind and heart. You may need to temporarily set aside many of the principles and patterns you've internalized. You may need to embrace a new definition of strength, one that doesn't always display itself in visible ways.

Chapter 10

Immediate:
Oneness & Meditation

Fruit. Ground. Cultivate.
— Grandmaster Yu

A few years ago, I had just delivered the first day of Oneness training to a friend named Thomas when he commented, "You're describing something that sounds similar to meditation. I've practiced meditation for about a year. How is it different from Oneness? How do you distinguish the two?"

I paused. How could I articulate in words the profound yet subtle difference between these two transformative practices? Both originated from Eastern wisdom traditions. Both emphasize the power of presence. Both offer proven paths to greater peace and well-being.

Thanks to the tremendous efforts of Dr. Jon Kabat-Zinn, a renowned American medical doctor, bestselling author, and teacher who developed Mindfulness Based Stress Reduction (MBSR), meditation has been integrated over the past few decades into conventional medicine and healthcare in the Western world. Science has validated its effectiveness for reducing stress, combatting pain, developing focus, and enhancing emotional regulation.

So, let me say it again: There is no doubt that meditation is a powerful tool. I have immense respect for loyal practitioners.

Nevertheless, there are fundamental differences between meditation and Oneness—which I have experienced personally.

In meditation, the observer stance creates space between you and your experience, allowing you to respond rather than react to life's ups and downs. It is a wonderful exercise. And I believe that Oneness allows you to go deeper.

After several minutes, I came up with this analogy to share with Thomas: "Picture yourself standing on the banks of a powerful river. The water rushes past, carrying leaves, twigs, and occasional flashes of light as the sun catches the ripples. In traditional meditation practice, you are the observer on the riverbank. You notice the river's movements without judgment. You witness your thoughts, emotions, and sensations as they flow by, neither clinging to them nor pushing them away."

"In Oneness practice, something more profound happens," I continued. "You don't remain standing on the riverbank as a separate observer. Instead, you enter the river. You become the water itself—flowing, powerful, interconnected with everything. You experience the energy of the current not as something separate from you, but as your very essence."

The next day, Thomas returned for further training. He already had a good grasp of the basic Oneness standing posture—shoulders relaxed back, slight smile, gentle gaze, feet firmly rooted. But his brows wrinkled and his body remained tense.

"I can watch my thoughts like clouds passing in the sky," he said. "Thanks to meditating for this past year, I've gotten pretty good at not getting caught up in them. But the same thing happens when I practice Oneness as when I meditate. I still feel frustrated. I don't understand what I'm supposed to be doing: Observing my bodily sensations? Focusing on my breath? What should I be aware of?"

"You're still asking questions like a meditation practitioner," I smiled. "Remember the analogy I shared with you: In Oneness, we don't observe the river—we become it. Stop trying to watch your experience and simply *be* your experience."

Thomas looked confused but determined. "Okay. I'll try."

A few minutes passed. Then something remarkable happened. The strained expression vanished from Thomas's face. His body appeared both solid and fluid at once, like a branch of bamboo that could bend in the wind without breaking.

At the end of the session, tears streamed down his cheeks. "I get it! I feel it! I've been watching the river for nearly a year. Today, for the first time, I became the river."

Fruit First

Perhaps the most revolutionary aspect of Oneness practice as compared to meditation is what Grandmaster Yu calls the "fruit first" approach. "Meditation is *cause, ground, cultivate*. Oneness is *fruit, ground, cultivate*," he says.

What does he mean?

Traditional meditation follows a cause-based model. You begin with discipline (the cause), and gradually work toward peace, clarity, and presence (the result). It's like planting a seed and nurturing it with consistent water and sunlight until, eventually, it bears fruit. This path often requires years of dedicated practice before experiencing profound results.

Oneness flips this model completely upside-down. Instead of starting with the cause and working toward the result, you begin with the result itself. The moment you stand in the Oneness posture, with your body aligned and a smile on your face, energy begins to flow. You don't have to practice for years in order to enjoy the benefits because you embody them from the very first moment.

"But how is that possible?" my students often ask. "How can I experience the result before I've done the work?"

I explain it this way: Oneness isn't something you need to create—it's your natural state. It's what you experience when you remove the blocks to your essential nature. The standing posture, with its precise alignment and openness, establishes the conditions whereby these blocks naturally dissolve.

This is why many Oneness practitioners report feeling immediate benefits, even in their first session. The fruit—that sense of unity, energy flow, and presence—is available right away. And as practice continues, it only deepens and expands.

The Power of the Posture

Other critical differences between meditation and Oneness practice help to explain why Oneness is "fruit first."

Standing posture

Generally speaking, you meditate while seated with your eyes closed. This creates a kind of inner sanctuary from which to observe your experience. You then aim to tame your "monkey mind" by telling it to quiet down. But the mind analyzing the mind creates an endless loop of thinking about thinking, which can prove frustrating even for many advanced meditation practitioners.

When you start with the body in Oneness, you bypass this loop. Grandmaster Yu says, "We correct the mind through the body." As you stand in the proper posture, energy begins to circulate throughout your body in ways you can actually feel. You experience warmth, tingling, pulsing, and flowing sensations almost immediately. As in meditation, you may continue to experience "monkey mind," but the energy of your body helps you return to the present moment.

Subtle smile

Practicing Oneness with a subtle smile also serves as a physiological key that unlocks a different state of being. Research from Stanford University has confirmed what ancient wisdom has always known: The simple act of smiling changes your biochemistry, shifting you from the contracted state of self-protection to the expanded state of openness and connection.

Eyes wide open

Furthermore, practicing with your eyes open in Oneness might seem like a small detail, but it represents a fundamental philosophical difference. With meditation, the primary focus is on developing your internal awareness—the ability to observe your thoughts, emotions, and sensations with clarity and without judgment. Such a practice is invaluable, especially in our culture where we're often disconnected from our inner experience.

But keeping your eyes closed subtly reinforces your sense of separation from the world. Opening your eyes helps dissolve this boundary, allowing you to remain connected to your environment while experiencing deep internal stillness. With Oneness, you rapidly move beyond self-awareness to selflessness. You don't deny yourself, but rather view yourself as inseparable from everything around you. The boundary between "in here" and "out there" softens and eventually dissolves.

In this expanded state, problems that once seemed overwhelming begin to reveal their solutions. Creativity flows more freely. Relationships deepen. Life itself becomes less of a struggle and more of a gentle float down the river.

The Value of an Empty Cup

"Empty your mind of all thoughts, let your heart be at peace," the *Tao Te Ching* advises. "In the pursuit of knowledge, something is added every day. In the practice of the Tao, every day something is dropped. When nothing is done, nothing is left undone."

I've found this wisdom to be the cornerstone of my Oneness practice. The greatest obstacles to our well-being are not external forces such as the stress of work or caretaking, unreasonable demands on our time, or even mental illness and chronic pain. The greatest obstacle is the Self, the ego. Our biases, fears, and concerns literally constrain our bodies and minds, leading to disease and unhappiness.

As you practice Oneness, you gradually let go of the Self, releasing accumulated knowledge and ego. You shed the constraints that used to limit you. This gentle psychological process of release allows your body's inherent wisdom to emerge, naturally enabling you to tap into your profound energy and internal power.

This inner power becomes a way of living in harmony with the world, embodying the principle of non-doing in every aspect of your life. When you achieve this state of alignment, you tap into a wellspring of energy and wisdom that can heal, enlighten, and empower in ways that transcend conventional understanding.

Chapter 11

Stress-free:
Oneness & Biohacking

Why do you need other exercise? Oneness is enough.
— Grandmaster Yu

Living in the San Francisco Bay Area over these past few years, I have encountered several people who are obsessed with biohacking. Over lunch at a recent conference, I listened as a woman in her mid-30s detailed her extensive regimen. It involved ice baths at precisely 39 degrees several times a week, a meticulously timed regimen of protein and supplements along with a total dedication to avoiding carbs and sugar, and data-driven exercise protocols designed to maximize mitochondrial function. I was astonished to learn that she even tracked her sleep.

Her passion was evident, her knowledge of the human body impressive. Yet beneath her enthusiasm, I noticed something else: Exhaustion. Her pursuit of physical and mental optimization had become yet another source of stress.

"Have you ever considered that all this effort might be working against you?" I asked gently.

The woman laughed. "I have," she replied. "It's a lot."

Since she had demonstrated openness to a conversation about Oneness, I explained how taking a fundamentally different approach to health and vitality had healed me from numerous physical ailments, including chronic pain and asthma, and had also alleviated my anxiety. I watched as her attitude shifted from curiosity to a genuine interest in learning more about this simple and ancient practice.

The Battle to Take Control

When we examine modern fitness culture, particularly the biohacking movement, we see an approach built on intervention, optimization, and control. It's about pushing the body to its limits, measuring every variable, and manipulating internal systems to achieve predetermined outcomes.

While impressive in its scientific sophistication, this approach often misses something essential about how our bodies naturally function and heal. Proper exercise should stimulate cellular renewal and enhance physical strength while supporting overall wellbeing. It should leave you feeling energized rather than depleted.

Yet many conventional forms of exercise and the latest and greatest biohacking protocols being touted by health and longevity influencers actually create stress on the bodily system. They cause the heart to overwork before muscles are fully warmed up, lead to rapid breathing, spike cortisol levels, and disrupt our natural recovery processes.

As with the woman I met at the conference, the real difficulty for most people living in our fast-paced modern world is that biohacking adds to our stress by placing even more demands on us. People who adopt this methodology are constantly striving to be perfect, to keep up with the latest research and techniques, to push themselves further without ever relaxing into life.

And then, when they slip up—which we all do, as human beings—they spiral into self-criticism, beating themselves up for not doing enough, not being enough.

Is this approach really helpful?

Strength Without Strain

Oneness offers a radically different approach.

Rather than forcing the body into submission through external intervention, Oneness practice creates conditions whereby your natural vitality can emerge from within. In contrast, biohacking often requires significant effort, expense, and continuous adjustment of variables. Exhaustion frequently follows these intense regimens.

The beauty of Oneness lies in its simplicity. Though the stationary postures appear to require minimal effort, they actually stimulate the body internally, strengthening muscles and organs, and promoting balanced growth across the entire system. Gradually, your body enters into a deeply regenerative state without creating stress.

The idea that Oneness supports internal cellular repair and energy regulation is backed up by thousands of years of traditional Chinese medical wisdom. When you operate in harmony with nature, small, controlled movements and even complete stillness can yield health benefits more profound than the most cutting-edge interventions.

The Oneness Diet

One of the most beautiful aspects of Oneness is its adaptability to different body types and circumstances. Whether standing, sitting, or lying down, all variations follow the same core principles: non-doing, non-judging, and non-attaching. When we practice Oneness, the energy and awareness generated naturally reset our bodies, creating a foundation of well being that transforms every aspect of life.

For many people, this integration extends into how we nourish ourselves. As my practice deepened, I naturally began eating more healthfully and mindfully. I slowed down, truly tasting and appreciating my food. I craved food that comes directly from the earth most of all.

And yet even so, in my experience, foods that might cause issues for other people—such as carbs and sugar—often don't create problems for dedicated Oneness practitioners. For example, I enjoy eating some meat and plenty of whole grains, fruit and vegetables. These food groups make up the majority of my diet. But when I want to, I consume sweets and treats without stressing about it. I trust my body, and it works. Lab tests measuring my cholesterol, diabetes markers, and other indicators consistently show that I am in excellent health.

When we align with our body's natural intelligence through Oneness practice, we often find that strict biohacking protocols become unnecessary. The body has its own innate wisdom about what it needs and doesn't need, which we can tap into. We sleep more deeply, digest more efficiently, and move through the world with greater ease.

Oneness is Enough

When Grandmaster Yu's students ask if they can continue activities like running and weight lifting alongside their Oneness practice, he smiles and says, "Sure, you can. But why do you need other exercise? Oneness is enough."

His response is not intended to dismiss any activity that you enjoy practicing, but rather to invite you to discover the completeness that Oneness offers.

When I first encountered these principles, they seemed too good to be true. How could something so simple address the complex health challenges I faced? But as I experienced healing in my own body, I realized that simplicity isn't a limitation—it is the ultimate sophistication.

Oneness truly is a one-stop shop for energy, awareness, and wisdom. It can serve as a complete practice in itself, or as a foundation that enhances everything else in your life. You do not need to choose between Oneness and other approaches. Please, keep up with any activities you enjoy. Just allow yourself to discover what helps your unique body to thrive with the least amount of struggle and the greatest amount of joy.

Chapter 12

Your True Nature

At this stage, you're not doing Oneness; you're living it.

Elena, an attorney and single mother in her late 40s, was new to Oneness. But she had been practicing mindfulness for several years. At the end of the first day of our training, it was clear that something was troubling her.

"What's going on?" I asked.

"I feel such peace when I practice mindfulness," she confessed, "but the moment I step back into my daily life—dealing with my teenage son, navigating conflicts at work—I leave that peace behind. It's as if my practice and my life exist in two separate worlds. How do I bridge that gap with Oneness?"

Many people compartmentalize their spiritual practices, treating them as sacred activities separate from the messiness of everyday existence. They sit silently for an hour each morning, then spend the rest of the day rushing, worrying, and reacting just like everyone else.

"The real magic of Oneness is that it impacts every aspect of your life, transforming how you engage with the world," I replied. "The key is not suppressing negative emotions or forcing a particular state, but rather bringing the quality of awareness, open heartedness, and effortless energy that is cultivated in your Oneness practice into your everyday experience."

After another week, Elena reported back to me that Oneness was helping. She had noticed subtle shifts in how she was able to navigate challenging situations at work and at home.

"I was in a contentious negotiation yesterday," she shared. "Normally, I would have met aggression with aggression, tensing up and pushing back. But something different happened. I felt a sensation of spaciousness open up inside me, just like what happens when I'm standing still. Instead of reacting, I was able to pause and respond with a clarity that I've never experienced before. I even smiled! The whole dynamic of the negotiation shifted, and we reached a resolution that benefited everyone."

I've witnessed similar transformations in countless students. The executive who no longer erupts in anger during stressful meetings. The parent who responds with patience rather than reactivity to a child's tantrum. The artist who moves through creative blocks with curiosity rather than frustration.

What is Natural?

In today's world, when you are led astray by habitual tendencies—whether that be stewing in anger and resentment, berating yourself for your supposed failures, or indulging in drinking, medications, gambling, shopping, or watching TikTok videos—you may feel that you are taking the easier path in life.

But the truth is, you are making life harder for yourself. Why? Because you are deviating from what is natural. "Natural" means alignment with nature. Our true nature corresponds with reason and the inherent order of things. It is not passive or irresponsible, but rather proactive. In the Taoist view, when a person is calm, they are naturally aligned with their inherent state.

When you practice Oneness, you rediscover what it is like to be in touch with nature. You relax physically and mentally. Without effort, you begin to let go of striving and attachments. You embrace the Way, the essence of life.

To attain this natural state, it helps to remain free from distractions for extended periods of time. Then, the wisdom of your body emerges and a clear state of mind surfaces, which results in an open heart.

If you stand in your natural state for just five minutes, as taught in Oneness, you soon will find yourself curiously unaffected by external forces. The longer and more frequently you practice, the more easily this effortless state will arise. If external forces try to intrude, your body either absorbs or neutralizes them, ensuring balance is maintained. Through consistent practice, you will flow like water along a rocky stream bed, adapting to any situation with ease.

Within just a few weeks or months, depending on how regularly you practice Oneness, you will discover that you can stay centered through even the greatest challenges of life. Whether you lose your job, get in a fight with a family member, suffer the pain of an illness, or struggle to make ends meet financially, you will be able to harness the limitless vitality of the world around you.

Many practitioners of Oneness talk about how they're able to tap into the joyful flow of life's energy for the first time since they were young children. Very little infiltrates this inner peaceful state.

Coming Home

In our complex, fast-paced world, we are conditioned to believe that effective solutions must be equally complex. Yet Oneness reveals a counterintuitive truth: The simplest approach often leads to the most profound results.

Oneness brings us home to our true nature.

This doesn't mean the journey is always easy. Cultivating a state of open heartedness and mental clarity requires consistent effort, especially at first. It is like water—if kept at a steady temperature, it remains calm and harmonious. If disrupted, it boils over or freezes, losing its natural flow.

The journey begins with a structured daily practice that builds a solid foundation. Here, the goal is to maintain a balanced, fluid state. Gradually, this state expands. Over time, new habits replace old, chaotic patterns, creating a steady and contemplative existence.

Even as you become advanced in your practice, you will not reach a destination once and for all. Yet even so, as your practice deepens, everything you do—from eating a meal, to having a conversation, to managing a meeting—becomes a doorway to presence. At this stage, you're not *doing* Oneness; you're *living* it.

PART IV

The Practice
of Oneness

Chapter 13

What to Expect

There is a logical progression to Oneness.

Now that you understand where it comes from and how Oneness can heal, it's time to learn how to do it correctly. In this part, I lay out a step-by-step approach to the practice.

If you have read the book up to this point, by now you most likely have high expectations of what Oneness can do for you. On the contrary, if you skipped ahead from the Introduction straight to this part of the book, then you may be approaching Oneness with skepticism.

That's okay. I've been there. No matter how you're feeling at this moment, all you have to do is give it a try and see if Oneness works for you.

Since Oneness is rooted in the Taoist concept of non-doing or *wu wei*, I encourage you to let go of the Self and trust your body to heal itself naturally. It's best not to force outcomes or obsess over achieving predetermined goals. Instead, allow space for your natural vitality to emerge.

Here are some key pointers:

- **Commit to start:** Set yourself a goal of practicing every day for at least a month, even if just for five minutes at a time. Consistency matters more than duration of practice, especially in the beginning.

- **Find your optimal time:** The morning, just after waking and completing your bathroom routine, offers the perfect opportunity to practice before the day's demands begin. That said, a different time might work better for you. Choose what suits you best. Just be sure to schedule in your Oneness practice as a non-negotiable part of your day.
- **Create space:** Wear comfortable, loose-fitting clothing and find a quiet place where you won't be disturbed. You may practice indoors or outdoors.
- **Honor your natural pace:** When you begin, you might only stand for 5 minutes. That is perfectly fine. Gradually increase to 10 minutes, then 15 minutes, listening to your body's wisdom. Enjoy the practice without pushing yourself too hard. The goal isn't to endure discomfort, but rather to discover comfort within the practice.
- **Welcome changes:** After a few days of consistent practice, you'll likely start feeling genuine joy during your practice time. You may also notice physical sensations—perhaps discomfort in areas that need healing, or tingling, warmth, and even gentle shaking in your hands, feet, or other parts of your body. These are often positive signs that energy is beginning to flow, sometimes revealing tensions you didn't even know you were carrying. Let them arise and pass without becoming overly attached to any sensation, positive or negative.
- **Develop a ritual:** Over time, your practice will transform from a discipline into a ritual. It will become something you look forward to each day. You'll also notice subtle improvements in your health, mood, and energy. Your family might comment on the changes in your presence before you even recognize them yourself. Allow it all without judgment.

No Perfect Posture

The great masters emphasize that the specific form or posture is not the most important aspect of Oneness practice. Each human body is different. Instead of struggling to rigidly adhere to a "perfect" posture, focus instead on finding the position that allows your body, with all its unique strengths and challenges, to completely relax.

This approach to Oneness encourages understanding the *why* behind the practice, rather than just mimicking a specific form. When you grasp the principles, you can adapt the practice to your needs, ensuring you receive its full benefits.

Trust the process.

Chapter 14

Why Guidance Matters

Traveling the simplest path requires clear directions,
especially when that path leads us home to ourselves.

I thought long and hard about it, and ultimately decided not to include any photos or illustrations in this book. It's true: The postures are incredibly simple. You will be inclined to mimic them right away in order to get started. Yet when it comes to self-study, several challenges present themselves.

In the modern world, most of us are consumed by stress and full of hidden tensions. We require the assistance of a trainer to identify how to relax. And even then, with Oneness, you don't relax completely in a sluggish way, as when collapsing onto the sofa to watch TV. Rather, you maintain an energetic posture.

The concept of non-doing challenges us at our core because it contradicts everything our society has conditioned us to value. We're taught from a young age that progress only comes through hard work, that results require striving, that achievement demands action. But if we complicate Oneness practice with such efforts, we disrupt the natural flow, leading to stagnation rather than progress.

As a result, reaching a state of true relaxation—wherein both body and mind release completely into presence—isn't something most of us can discover alone, especially when beginning this practice. It is paradoxical. You must relax into the art of non-doing while also paying attention to subtle shifts in your body position and mind.

As Grandmaster Wang Xiangzhai emphasized, "In the study of the method of standing, the most important thing is to avoid exerting ourselves, either mentally or physically. If we use physical strength, our energy (Qi), will be congested and blocked. When our Qi is blocked, our intention (Yi), is stopped. When our intention is blocked, our spirit (Shen), will be distracted. And when our spirit is distracted, we will be deluded into thinking we're making progress when actually we're regressing."

This is precisely where guidance becomes not just helpful but essential for most people.

You might find yourself questioning, "If Oneness is really as simple and direct as you say, then why do I need guidance from a coach?"

Even though the method is straightforward, every single person will experience different changes and challenges along the way. Your body holds its own unique patterns of tension, shaped by your life experiences, injuries, and emotional history. Your mind has its particular tendencies and obstacles. As you practice, unexpected sensations, emotions, or insights typically emerge, which leave you wondering: *Is this normal? Am I doing this right? Should I continue?*

This is why I strongly encourage you to attend a low-cost, in-person training session if you can.

The Role of the Sensei

When I found my sensei, Grandmaster Yu, I had a breakthrough early on. During a practice session, he circled me as I stood in the basic posture. "You're holding tension here," he said, barely touching my right shoulder. "And here," his fingers brushed my lower back. "And especially here," he noted, hovering his hand near my jaw.

I hadn't noticed any of it. These patterns of tension had become so familiar that they were invisible to me. They were like the background noise of sirens and honking horns that you stop hearing after living in a busy city for a few months.

A certified coach or sensei can help you relax, identifying where in your body and mind you are still carrying tension. They can adjust your posture to ensure that you're benefiting as much as possible. Your coach can also help to explain the *why* of Oneness first, and then the *how*, and follow with teaching the stages in a logical progression. They will clarify, accelerate, and deepen your healing process.

You can also join an online training program. But even online, coaches are limited in not being able to observe your body from all angles or feel your energy. Most students report that attending an in-person training is the most effective method.

Of course, this book is here to instruct you in the fundamental principles, history, and reasons why Oneness works. In addition, you can go to the Oneness Institute website or YouTube channel and watch some videos of me training in order to get a sense of what's involved. Nevertheless, your practice will be greatly enhanced with individual guidance.

During your journey, having someone with you who has walked the path before you is invaluable. They recognize the landmarks, understand the territory, and can reassure you when you're headed in the right direction—or gently redirect you when you've strayed from the path. A good sensei or coach will catalyze breakthroughs that might otherwise take you years to achieve—or simply end with you giving up.

As with martial arts, the relationship between student and teacher in Oneness practice goes deeper than conventional coaching. This is why I prefer the term *sensei* to *coach*. A coach tends to focus primarily on technique and performance. A sensei walks the path alongside you, communicating with you at a deeper level, helping you navigate not just the practice but the life transformation it catalyzes.

Finding Your Guide

When seeking guidance for your Oneness practice, look beyond credentials and charisma. Instead, notice how you feel in your coach or sensei's presence. Do they embody the qualities that drew you to this practice? Most importantly, have they been transformed by Oneness themselves?

The finest teachers don't position themselves as the source of your healing, but instead help you connect with the healing capacity already within you. They have no desire to carry you across the river because they want you to discover that you already know how to swim.

As you continue your Oneness journey, remember that seeking guidance is not a sign of weakness, but rather a symbol of your own wisdom. Even the most accomplished practitioners continue to benefit from the perspective and insights that a skilled guide can offer. Traveling the simplest path requires clear directions, especially when that path leads us home to ourselves.

Chapter 15

Begin Your Journey Today

This book is your map.

Imagine you hold in your hands a beautiful map. It is detailed, precise. It shows spectacular mountains, rivers, forests, and valleys. You can trace the paths with your fingertip and envision what it must feel like to stand at the summit of the peak or beside a flowing river.

The map gives you clarity. It allows you to see where you are and where you could go. You understand the landscape from a distance. You have an intellectual understanding, a mindful awareness of what is out there.

This book is your map.

But then, you put down the map and take your first step. You feel the roughness of the stones beneath your feet. You smell the pine in the air. You hear the rush of a hidden stream. The wind brushes against your skin. You taste the freshness of wild berries that you pick as you walk past.

This is what happens when you actually begin to practice Oneness. You're not studying the map anymore—you're hiking the landscape. Every sense awakens. Every cell in your body becomes part of the landscape. You are within it, and it is within you.

The map, this book, is a guide. But now you are the traveler, the path, and the destination all at once. You move beyond *knowing* the way to *being* the way.

ONENESS

Oneness is not about striving. All you have to do is stand still and settle in. When you stop *forcing* and start *allowing*, stop *doing* and enjoy *being,* you merge with the energy of the universe. Instead of draining your batteries, you recharge them effortlessly.

Take the first step on your journey today, so that you can begin to experience the miracle of this ancient and simple practice for yourself as soon as possible.

Chapter 16

Stage 1: Reset & Recovery

*Its simplicity tricks many people into thinking
that Oneness is foolish.*

Its simplicity tricks many people into thinking that Oneness is foolish.

Even my wife was skeptical of Oneness for several years after I began to practice daily. She watched me, saying, "Sure, LD, that's fine for you. But I prefer to exercise." Then she would set off for the pool, where she devotedly swam laps every day.

Over time, however, she noticed my personality was changing. "You're calmer," she commented. "I feel like you're a different person. Where's your temper?"

I just smiled. "Oneness," I said.

Then, about two years ago, she began to experience symptoms of menopause, including insomnia and constipation.

"Oneness," I suggested with a grin.

"Okay fine, I'll try it," she consented with a sigh of frustration.

After just two days of practice, she slept soundly through the night. No more than a week had gone by before she declared that her constipation was no more. "I can't believe it. How is it possible that just standing still can do so much?" she remarked.

Now, my wife practices Oneness twice a day every day. She is as much of a believer as I am.

The simplicity of Oneness is not foolish. In fact, Grandmaster Yu teaches the exact opposite: Adding extra details is foolish. Why make things more complex? You'll only make it less likely that people will stick with the practice.

The Simplest Start

Scan the internet and you'll find multiple examples of people who have lifted cars with their bare hands in feats of extraordinary strength in order to save the life of their child, parent, or even a stranger. Later, they're unable to repeat this task. This example demonstrates that your body has immense potential to harness the energy that exists within us and in nature all the time. And that potential is far greater than most people ever imagine.

You simply need the right conditions to unlock and fully release your potential.

In the modern world, most people's minds are full of stress and worries, their bodies full of tension. When they come to Oneness, they often feel weak, anxious, depressed, and depleted. Hence, they lack sufficient energy to follow a regular program of fitness, meditation, or self-improvement—or even to simply enjoy their lives.

Stage 1 of Oneness is the perfect place to begin to counter these limitations.

The simplest standing posture offers the easiest, most minimal effort. It is so minimalist, in fact, that you can't even really tell if someone is practicing Oneness or not. It looks like doing nothing! The only difference is that after practicing for some time, you will find your stress levels reduced, your energy levels boosted, and your awareness increased.

If you jump to Stage 2 or 3, which involves raising your arms, you will create extra tension in your shoulders and chest, preventing you from relaxing fully. And in fact, if you are still stressed out, it won't work for you to mimic the more advanced postures. Instead, start at Stage 1 with your arms relaxed by your side.

Stage 1 Practice

The posture design is truly genius. It is intended to be effortless. Like an old-school radio, when you tune to the right frequency, the static clears and the signal comes in without interference.

Inside our bodies, there are hidden "switches." When we switch on, tension releases and circulation, breath, energy and awareness flow more freely.

There is a top-down chain. It begins by softening the space between your eyebrows. This gentle release sends a signal of safety that helps your brain ease out of stress mode. From there, the impact cascades downward. Your chest loosens. Your heart feels lighter. Your breath naturally deepens. Your whole body relaxes.

It's a body-to-brain shortcut. A small physical shift that interrupts stress loops and invites the parasympathetic system back online. This is the branch of the nervous system that restores calm and balance.

The 9 Switches

Here are the 9 hidden switches in your body that you will turn on when you practice Stage 1 of Oneness.

- **Switch 1: Crown Lift**
Your spinal cord is the main highway of energy through your body. The main corridor of your nervous system. Straightening your spine is the crown lift switch.

Imagine a silk thread gently lifting you from the crown of your head, so that your head floats. This happens without force. Your spine lengthens slightly as you stack your vertebrae taller.

Standing upright in this way lightens the disc load, especially as compared to sitting slumped over your phone or computer. Research reveals that unsupported or slumped sitting increases lumbar intradiscal pressure by 40% versus upright standing.

When your spine is aligned, neurological signals travel without unnecessary mechanical stress.

- **Switch 2: Eyes & Ears**

Your eyes and ears serve as the switch for panoramic awareness. Connection with nature expands and fear dissipates.

Look forward horizontally, as if staring at a distant horizon. Do not look down. Expand your view to 180 degrees. Listen behind you, as well. Together, that's 360 degrees of awareness. Feel yourself immersed in nature.

Research shows that stress tends to narrow our attentional focus. Adopting a broader field of awareness reduces arousal.

In this state, your body feels safe. The red alert of stress and anxiety turns off.

- **Switch 3: Smile**

This switch turns on your brain's relaxation channel.

Smile gently from the heart, turning your corners of your lips upward. Keep your mouth slightly open, with your tongue resting lightly on the roof. Soften the space between your eyebrows. Let an easy, slight look of happiness spread from your face across the rest of your body.

Scientific research reveals that smiling triggers a biochemical cascade across our bodies. Our muscles release and calmness spreads. When smiling with a slightly open mouth, breathing deepens naturally, the nervous system downshifts, energy flows deeper, and the mind quiets. Meta-analysis of numerous studies show that smiling speeds cardiovascular recovery from stress and reduces cortisol levels.

• Switch 4: Feet & Knees

This is your grounding spring base, enabling your body to carry you effortlessly.

Stand with your feet shoulder-width apart or narrower, but not wider. Distribute your weight evenly, or a bit more towards the heels. Bend your knees slightly. Never lock them, and never bend them so far that your knees go past your toes.

Shake your body gently up and down. Then pause at the upward point, knees soft. This slight knee flexion engages the limb "springs," improving your balance and shock absorption, according to scientific research.

• Switch 5: Pelvic Tuck

This switch is your core stabilizer. It supports balance and breath.

Tuck your pelvis slightly, as though you were sitting on a tall bar stool. This anchors your breath low in your belly even as your crown stays lifted. As a result, your spine becomes upright yet loose.

Research reveals that coordinated diaphragm-abdominal activation increases lumbar stability and reduces pressure on the spine.

• Switch 6: Shoulders & Chest

This switch activates your upper body release, freeing the heart and lungs.

Open your chest slightly, then let it return to a neutral position where it is neither caved in nor puffed out. Let your arms hang freely, as if disconnected from your shoulders. Maintain a small space between your arms and the trunk of your body, helping your shoulders to relax.

Scientific research shows that this neutral chest alignment supports breathing fully. This can reduce your risk of stroke and lower your heart rate.

- **Switch 7: Tiger's Mouth Hands**

This posture switches on the hand channel and melts tension from the shoulders.

Open your palms fully, fingers straight. Then loosen your hands and let the fingers return to a natural, slightly bent position. Keep the web between the thumb and index finger open. In Chinese, we call this hand position the Tiger's Mouth.

Research shows that over a period of weeks, isometric training in exercises such as hand grips lowers resting blood pressure. Reducing gripping effort and supporting the forearms reduces tension all the way up the chain to the shoulders.

Use the Tiger's Mouth cue to encourage that relaxation.

- **Switch 8: Whole-Body Stillness**

This switch is the master tuner that resets your whole system. With your posture lifted, your spirit rises. At the same time, as your muscles soften and your breath deepens, and your stress levels fall.

Allow your body to settle into proper alignment. Your head floats upward as if weightless. Your spine stretches tall, yet stays loose. Your lower back lifts slightly, supported by the pelvic tuck. Your knees rest soft and unlocked with a gentle upward spring.

Your posture is neither stiff nor slouched. Your head, lower back, and knees all lift gently upward. Meanwhile your muscles drop, shoulders fall, arms hang, and breath deepens. It's as though your body was an outfit hung on the hanger of your bone.

Blood pressure can rise when you hold a posture for a long time, so progress sensibly if you suffer from hypertension. But research demonstrates that attentional and stillness training brings about functional changes in your neural networks, effectively reducing default-mode activity.

- **Switch 9: Top-Down Scan**

The top-down scan switch polishes every signal. It is like the fine-tuning knob on old-fashioned radios that you turned slowly and carefully back and forth until the music came through crystal clear.

Sweep through your body with your mind, relaxing every part. Body-scan practices reduce stress, heart rate, and mind wandering, studies show.

Stage 1 Benefits

When all nine switches have been activated, your body becomes like a perfectly tuned radio—clear, resonant, and free of static. You might also think of it like a living orchestra. Each part is in harmony, and your whole body as one instrument. At that moment, you simply let it flow.

"Wow, this practice is truly fascinating," you may be thinking.

But, what you've done so far is not the practice yet, it's only the preparation, now, please stay with the posture, leave these behind, not stick to these details, and to enjoy

The Practice

Look forward toward the horizon, 180 degrees, Don't look down. Listen back 180 degrees, If you're outdoors, you may hear birds singing. Receive it. Feel and enjoy being one with nature. After a while, check in on your body. Relax your chest, lower back, and shoulders. If tension returns, smile again, soften again, sigh gently and let your breath drop.

It's so simple! Now you understand why I translate this practice as Oneness.

When all the switches are on, your body becomes a super-highway. Body and mind as one. A clear channel where energy and awareness flow freely. And you become one with nature. No striving. No trying. No need to force yourself to let go of anger, overthinking, stress or pain. You just let things come to you naturally. Through this non-doing, energy and awareness build up. The muddy water settles. Clarity appears on its own.

Then, the true you emerges. You discover the power of healing. You rest in peace, compassion,and love.

Sitting Practice

If you are disabled, elderly, or too sick to stand, sitting is a viable alternative. You can also practice Oneness from a seated position whenever you find yourself in a meeting, riding in a vehicle, or sitting on a plane. The same principles apply in all these scenarios.

The sitting posture is as follows:

- Sit upright and still.
- Chair: Ensure the chair height is slightly higher than your knees.
- Feet: Position your feet shoulder-width apart or slightly narrower. They can either lay flat on the floor or you can keep your heels on the floor and your toes pointed slightly upwards.
- Hips: Sit with your hips only halfway on the chair.
- Waist: Relax your waist.
- Chest: Open your chest.
- Shoulders: Relax your shoulders.
- Arms: Let your arms drop naturally and lay flat on the tops of your thighs, near the knees.
- Neck: Relax your neck.
- Mouth: Open your mouth slightly and smile gently.
- Chin: Keep your chin slightly tucked.

- Eyes: Look straight ahead, without focusing on anything.
- Alignment: Follow the guidelines as the standing posture, ensuring that your body remains relaxed and aligned, allowing energy to flow freely.

Laying Down Practice

If you can't practice while standing or sitting due to a physical disability, sickness, or other limitation, then you can practice Oneness while lying down. If you are able to practice standing but suffer from insomnia, you may want to do an additional session at night, while lying in bed. This will help you fall into a deep and restful slumber.

The lying down posture is as follows:

- Lie down flat on your back on a comfortable surface.
- Legs: Keep your legs slightly apart.
- Knees and feet: You can bend your knees to place your feet flat upon the floor, or straighten your knees and allow your toes to point upward.
- Hips: Allow your hips to relax.
- Waist: Relax your waist.
- Chest: Open your chest.
- Shoulders: Relax your shoulders.
- Arms: Lay your arms naturally at your sides, palms facing downward, or rest them on your abdomen.
- Neck: Relax your neck, keeping it aligned with your spine.
- Mouth: Open your mouth slightly and smile gently.
- Eyes: Look gently upwards, without focusing on anything.

- Alignment: Follow the same guidelines as the sitting posture, ensuring that your body remains relaxed and aligned, allowing energy to flow freely.

You may continue with Stage 1 practice for as long as you like.

Chapter 17

Stage 2: Cultivation

*In Stage 2, you focus on nurturing your body in
order to achieve greater strength and vitality.*

For beginners who are stressed out and feel tension and pain all
over their bodies, adding extra steps complicates Oneness practice
too much. It makes it more challenging for you to relax completely.
This is why I encourage you again to start practicing at Stage 1,
huifu, for some time before you move on.

There is no prescribed duration for you to continue before
advancing to Stage 2. The timing varies for each individual,
depending on your condition at the start of your Oneness journey and your commitment to the practice.

Over time, you'll notice your energy gradually increasing.
You may experience healing of illnesses and chronic pain, relief
from mental health struggles such as depression and anxiety, and
significant improvements in your interpersonal relationships.
You will feel an emerging sense of inner peace.

At this point, you may be ready for Stage 2.

Climbing the Mountain

Advancing through the stages of Oneness is rather like
climbing a mountain. Everyone knows that the view from the
summit is vast, breathlessly beautiful, and awe-inspiring. Yet few
people make it there.

When you start to climb, the view doesn't change much, even though you know you're ascending because your breathing is getting harder and you're sweating slightly. Many people quit right here, before they've even begun. They will never know the benefits of Oneness.

But if you stick with it, then once you climb to a certain level, maybe halfway up the mountain, you begin to enjoy a view out over the surrounding landscape. You feel excited. You might choose to stop here. Enjoy yourself! It's already wonderful, right?

This is Stage 1 of Oneness. If healing is your only goal, then a Stage 1 practice may be sufficient for you. And that is perfectly acceptable.

Other people will not be satisfied, however. They want to climb higher, knowing they will enjoy even better views. That said, the only way to continue is to gather more energy, more resources. Make sure you drink plenty of water and eat a few snacks! In Stage 2 of Oneness, *peiyang*, you focus on nurturing your body in order to achieve greater strength and vitality.

The guidance and support of a coach is extremely helpful at this stage.

The Three Phases of Stage 2

The second stage actively engages your arms. This can introduce tension in the shoulders and chest, however. That is why, to avoid any issues, Stage 2 is divided into three progressive phases.

Phase 1

Stand as you did in Stage 1, but turn your hands so that your palms face upwards.

Hold this position for a while. If you experience no additional tension, then proceed to the next phase.

STAGE 2: CULTIVATION

Phase 2

Take it one step further by keeping the upper part of your arms relaxed while gently raising the lower part, from the elbows to the fingers. Hold your forearm and hands steady, parallel to the ground.

Once again, check for any added tension. If you still feel comfortable, then you can proceed to the next phase.

Phase 3

For this phase, raise the entire length of your arms, from the shoulders to the hands, to waist height. Hold them steady, parallel to the ground.

If no tension arises, you are engaging fully in Stage 2 of practice.

Chapter 18

Stage 3: Oneness

Oneness is limitless.

Congratulations, welcome to Stage 3!

After practicing Stage 2, *peiyang* or cultivation, for some time, your body should now be much more relaxed and generating even more energy. Once you can stand with your arms raised for extended periods without experiencing any added tension, you are ready for Stage 3, *hunyuan*.

To return to our mountain climbing analogy, you may now want to ascend to the summit. But unlike a mountain, which has a physical top, Oneness is limitless. It is always new. The views change constantly. Sometimes the sun shines, sometimes it is cloudy, but no matter what, you feel energized and content.

With your arms fully engaged, *hunyuan* brings your body into a state of dynamic balance. The strength of your muscles is not what helps you to raise your arms, but rather nature's flow.

Reaching Stage 3 is not necessary for everyone. But it is essential for cultivating greater awareness and can lead to spiritual awakening.

Transitioning to Hunyuan

All other aspects of the posture remain the same as in Stage 2, with the following adjustments:

- Arms: Begin by slowly raising your arms to a specific height between the belly button and the shoulders— no lower than the belly button, and no higher than the shoulders.
- Shoulders: Release any tension.
- Chest: Keep your chest relaxed.
- Hands: Turn your palms to face your chest, fingers extended.

Chapter 19

The Three Fists: A Complimentary Approach

These fists are not for fighting.

Three years ago, Grandmaster Yu Hongkun began teaching the ancient Chinese Three Fists method as a compliment to Oneness. He did this as a direct response to the greatest challenges he saw practitioners facing in today's world: Mental health issues, exhaustion, and burnout.

Whether practiced on its own or in combination with Stage 1, 2, or 3 of Oneness, the Three Fists method is a powerful way to boost energy, restore vitality, and cultivate inner joy. These days, Grandmaster Yu frequently has his students train in both techniques in one day. He has found that the combination of rest and release can create deep shifts from the inside out.

At first glance, the Three Fists method may resemble shadowboxing or martial arts. But don't be misled. In conventional boxing, punches are driven by your muscles. The physical action is meant to hit, defend, or win.

The Three Fists method is the opposite.

When you practice the Three Fists, you're not trying to hit anything. Instead, you're learning to release. The power doesn't come from your arm or shoulder muscles, but rather from your entire body working in harmony. You are rooted into the ground, aligned through the spine, expressing energy through your fists. All this happens without building up any tension.

Imagine a cannon firing. The cannon doesn't push the cannonball out, it simply releases it. The energy gathers from deep within and launches outward with one sudden, clean, powerful blast. That's exactly what happens when a fist is thrown in the Three Fists method. You don't use brute strength or try to generate power, but rather let go and allow power to emerge on its own. This restores your energy and combats burnout.

In order to work, your punches must be relaxed, not stiff. Released, not forced. And that's the real challenge—simply letting go.

These fists are not for fighting.

It is especially beneficial to have the guidance of a coach in order to master the Three Fists technique. The dynamic release can prove quite tricky for even the most advanced Oneness students to master. Also, your coach can work with you to determine how frequently and for how long you should focus on the Three Fists as a compliment to your personal Oneness program.

The Three Stages of The Three Fists

The Effortful Stage

In the beginning, most people unconsciously rely on muscle force to throw a punch. This is natural. But through steady practice with a coach, you can begin to release your fists. Embracing the principle of non-doing, your deeply ingrained habits of using force and effort begin to loosen.

The Forceless Stage

At this stage, you stop using force entirely. Your fists become soft. But they are not yet powerful. Here, you focus on refining your alignment, posture, and punch structure while continuing to let go.

THE THREE FISTS: A COMPLIMENTARY APPROACH

The Forceless Yet Powerful Stage

Eventually, when your alignment, structure, and awareness fully harmonize, the Three Fists becomes a practice that is at once both effortless and powerful. Energy flows freely throughout your body. You feel enlivened, awake, and stress-free.

Grandmaster Yu feels that complimenting your Oneness practice with the Three Fists is particularly beneficial if you are facing challenges to your mental health including depression, anxiety, extreme stress and/or burnout. In cases like these, when you feel totally sapped of energy, the Three Fists practice stimulates your energy and revives your vitality.

The Three Fists method is a living embodiment of the Oneness principle: In non-doing, everything is done.

Chapter 20

How Long Does It Take?

Bamboo grows roots for three years before blooming above ground. Every day you practice Oneness, you are growing roots.

Results from Oneness practice vary significantly depending on your health and mental condition when you start, whether you do in-person or online-only training sessions, how often you practice and for how long each day. Generally speaking, while some effects may be felt quickly, the deeper, long-term benefits unfold gradually with consistent practice. Oneness is a journey.

Most people report experiencing noticeable improvements in their energy level, quality of sleep, and overall sense of calm within just a few days, and significant improvements to their underlying health and psychological well-being within a few months. For severe conditions, it may take as long as a year to heal. In some cases, by committing to a sustained daily practice, people have even been known to cure themselves of cancer.

Grandmaster Yu says, "Oneness practice is like bamboo. Bamboo can take three years to establish a root system before sending visible shoots up above the ground. It can take five years to fully flourish. But then, bamboo grows at an astonishing rate of one to two feet per week. Even if noticeable changes seem delayed, your body begins transforming from the very first day of Oneness practice. It is growing its roots. One day soon, it will blossom."

ONENESS

To achieve the best results quickly, start with the right teaching, preferably in-person with an established coach or if not then online, and maintain a daily practice. From there, the key lies in your dedication—how much time you commit to the practice each day.

Over time, everything you do becomes an extension of Oneness, constantly bringing you closer to enlightenment and freedom.

Chapter 21

Navigating Common Challenges

Each moment of resistance, doubt, or difficulty offers a chance to deepen your understanding not just of the practice, but of yourself.

We live in a world that celebrates doing, striving, and visible achievements. Oneness invites us in the opposite direction—into stillness, presence, and the invisible power that emerges when we relax into what is so.

Here are some of the most common challenges you might encounter on this journey. I invite you to view them not as obstacles to overcome through force, but rather as doorways to step through with understanding and awareness.

The Impatience of Our Culture

"Shouldn't I feel something more? Is this even working?"

The most immediate challenge for some new practitioners is when they lack instant, tangible results. We've been conditioned by a culture that promises quick fixes for everything—take a pill for immediate pain relief, follow a 7-day diet for dramatic weight loss, download an app that promises transformation in 10 minutes a day.

Many people do experience benefits from Oneness starting with their very first practice session. With a slight smile on our faces, gazing out at the world with eyes open, we can sense energy flowing through us, uniting us with nature. We are enveloped in peace.

Nevertheless, the power of this ancient practice unfolds gradually, often beginning with subtle shifts beneath the surface of awareness. Beyond sensations of warmth, tingling, and calm, more profound benefits emerge only through consistent practice over weeks and even months. This can prove deeply unsettling to people accustomed to living in the fast-paced modern world. Doubts naturally arise.

The answer lies in patience. Trust the process. Oneness operates on its own timeline, not always the accelerated pace we've come to expect from technology. It's also critical to remind yourself that the deeper shifts in energy, awareness, and vitality often begin long before you consciously register them.

The Discomfort of Stillness

"I can't stand still for long. It's too hard."

I hear this complaint frequently, revealing how unaccustomed we've become to stillness. Many people discover that the simple act of standing without moving unveils tensions and imbalances they never knew they carried. Shoulders begin to ache, legs tremble, feet hurt, back muscles protest.

When uncomfortable physical sensations arise during practice, receive them not as problems to be eliminated but as messages to be received. Your body communicates years of accumulated stress and misalignment. Each discomfort represents an opportunity to release what no longer serves you. Each area of tension reveals where energy has been blocked, offering an opportunity for release and renewed flow. This shift in perspective transforms struggle into exploration.

Even more challenging than the physical discomfort for many people is the mental and emotional stillness that Oneness invites. Without the constant distractions of movement, screens, and activity, we come face-to-face with our thoughts and feelings. The mind races, worries surface, emotions arise.

In a culture that offers us endless ways to avoid our inner landscape, the invitation to be with whatever emerges can feel radical, frightening even. Yet it's precisely this willingness to be present that creates the space for genuine transformation.

The Fear of Losing Who We Think We Are

"What if I change too much? Will I still be me?"

This fear rarely gets expressed directly, yet I find that it underlies much of the resistance people experience to deepening their practice. Over time, Oneness shifts how you perceive yourself and the world. As you release tension and self-limiting beliefs, aspects of your identity that once seemed essential may begin to dissolve.

The ambitious executive who defined himself through achievement may discover a newfound contentment with simply being. The chronic worrier who couldn't sleep at night might find herself responding to life's challenges with unexpected ease. People who prided themselves on constant busy-ness might embrace periods of restful stillness.

These shifts can trigger a subtle identity crisis. The Ego, which maintains itself through familiar patterns and self-concepts, may resist the very changes that bring it greater peace and wellbeing. It prefers familiar discomfort to the unknown territory of freedom.

This resistance manifests itself as inconsistency in practice, sudden doubts about the validity of the method, or finding reasons why "this isn't the right time" to commit fully. When you notice these thought and behavior patterns arising, recognize them with compassion—then let them go. They're simply your mind clinging to what feels safe and known.

The Challenge of Non-Doing

"But where am I trying to get to? What will I achieve?"

At the heart of Oneness practice lies the principle of non-doing. Allowing rather than forcing. Receiving rather than grasping. Being rather than striving. While simple to understand intellectually, this concept can prove remarkably difficult to embody.

Ever since our caregivers cheered our very first steps in life, we've been rewarded for doing, achieving, and controlling outcomes. The suggestion that profound transformation might come through non-doing can seem not just counterintuitive, but almost threatening to our fundamental worldview.

Even if we're able to embrace the principle of non-doing on an intellectual level, our bodies and nervous systems have been conditioned for action. We instinctively tense muscles that could be relaxed, control breathing that could flow naturally, and mentally direct thought processes that would unfold more harmoniously without our interference.

One of the greatest challenges of many self-help and spiritual practices is to let go. With Oneness, we relax into it all, and so the letting go is effortless.

The Obstacles of Modern Life

Beyond these conceptual challenges lie the practical obstacles of modern life. Here are a few that might arise and impede your Oneness practice:

- **Problem:** *"I don't have time."*

This is perhaps the most common objection, yet it reveals a misunderstanding of what Oneness requires. Even five minutes of practice a day can shift your energy and awareness. The question isn't whether you have time, but whether you're willing to prioritize this form of self-care amidst competing demands.

Solution: Start with just five minutes.

Remove the time excuse immediately by committing to what I call "The 5-Minute Challenge." Stand in the basic posture for just five minutes each day for one week. Feel what happens in your body. Notice any subtle shifts in energy or awareness. Almost everyone can feel something change in just five minutes. That's enough to spark curiosity about continued practice.

Also, like me, you may very well find that Oneness gradually replaces many of your other activities, such as going to the gym and meditation. You actually end up with more time in the end.

- **Problem:** *"There are too many options out there."*

The wellness industry bombards us with countless methods promising transformation. Faced with an overwhelming array of choices—meditation apps, fitness programs, therapy modalities, spiritual practices, biohacking techniques—many people freeze in indecision or dabble superficially in multiple approaches without committing deeply to any.

- **Solution: Just try.**

Oneness is one for all. Along with many other Oneness practitioners, I have found it more effective in healing my mind and body than martial arts, meditation, traditional Chinese medicine, and many other activities that I tried. I urge you to try it for yourself. See if it works for you.

- **Problem: *"I can't disconnect."***

The constant pull of notifications, news, and social media has rewired our attention spans and created subtle addictions to stimulation. The prospect of standing quietly without digital distraction can trigger genuine withdrawal symptoms—restlessness, anxiety, and a physical craving for the next dopamine hit from our devices.

- **Solution: Reframe *boring* as *powerful*.**

When your mind labels stillness as boring, it's often protecting itself from deeper change. Consider that the most powerful forces in nature—gravity, electromagnetic fields, the growth of plants—operate invisibly and without drama. Your practice works the same way, generating power through stillness rather than obvious action.

Finding Your Way

If you recognize yourself in any of these challenges, know that you're not alone. Every sincere practitioner of Oneness encounters obstacles on the path, not because they're doing something wrong but because the practice itself is designed to reveal habits that limit our natural vitality.

The *Tao Te Ching* states, "When a superior scholar hears of the Tao, he diligently practices it. When a middling scholar hears of the Tao, he sometimes keeps it and sometimes loses it. When an inferior scholar hears of the Tao, he laughs loudly at it."

The simplicity of Oneness may seem almost laughable in a world that equates complexity and lightning speed with value. Yet in this very simplicity lies its profound power—the ability to return you to your natural state of harmony, balance, and flow. As you continue your journey with Oneness, remember that each moment of resistance, doubt, or difficulty offers a chance to deepen your understanding not just of the practice, but of yourself.

Chapter 22

Beyond Standing

*Your personal cultivation directly benefits
everyone you encounter.*

The ultimate goal of this practice isn't to become excellent at standing still. It is to embody the qualities of Oneness throughout your daily life.

Here are some practical strategies that have helped many people extend their practice beyond formal sessions:

1. Create micro-practices throughout your day.

Even thirty seconds of standing in the Oneness posture—perhaps before an important meeting, after a stressful phone call, or right before you go to sleep—can reset your nervous system and reconnect you with centered awareness.

2. Develop awareness of your body's signals.

Notice when tension begins to accumulate in your shoulders, jaw, or belly during challenging interactions. These physical cues often precede emotional reactivity. Simply recognizing and gently releasing this tension can prevent your stress from escalating.

3. Pause before responding.

In conversations, especially difficult ones, cultivate the habit of taking a breath before replying. This tiny gap creates space for wisdom to emerge instead of your automatic, highly charged emotional reactions.

4. View routine activities as part of your Oneness practice.

I never used to enjoy cleaning the house. But ever since becoming a regular practitioner of Oneness, I do my chores with genuine joy. I sing to myself as I mindfully cook dinner, wash the dishes, and make the bed. I smile and hum as I commute to work and wait in line at the grocery store. With Oneness, it feels quite natural to bring the same quality of relaxed awareness that you cultivate during your practice into your everyday activities.

5. Notice the impact of your presence.

Without becoming self-conscious, begin to observe how your internal state affects those around you. This awareness naturally motivates you to continue your practice, because it helps you recognize that your personal cultivation directly benefits everyone you encounter.

When you integrate Oneness into your everyday life, you don't need to announce each session to the world or create elaborate rituals or tell anyone that you're doing it. Simply allow it to become an invisible current flowing beneath all your activities, gradually transforming how you move through the world.

PART V

The Life of Oneness

Chapter 23

The Ripple Effect

The most radical aspect of Oneness isn't what it does for the individual practitioner, but how it ripples outward, changing families, workplaces, and communities.

The true measure of any spiritual practice lies not in what happens while we are doing it, but in how it transforms our engagement with the world. While the personal benefits of Oneness—which include improved health, mental clarity, and emotional balance—are profound, they represent only the beginning of its potential impact.

The most radical aspect of Oneness isn't what it does for the individual practitioner, but how it ripples outward, changing families, workplaces, and communities.

The Relationship Mirror

Our closest relationships often serve as the most sensitive barometers of our inner state. The tension we carry, the reactivity we harbor, and the fears we haven't addressed emerge most visibly in our interactions with our partners, children, and family members. As Oneness practice gradually unties these inner knots, your interpersonal relationships naturally transform.

My wife noticed the shift in me before I did. "You're more present," she told me about six months into my Oneness practice.

"When I'm talking to you, I feel like you're actually here, not just thinking about work."

This quality of presence is perhaps the most precious gift we can offer another human being. And it emerges naturally, as Oneness dissolves the preoccupations and stresses that typically pull us away from the present moment. When we're no longer constantly distracting ourselves, processing the past or planning for the future, we can truly *be*—not just with ourselves, but also with those we love.

Many students report similar transformations. Lily described how her relationship with her teenaged daughter shifted after she began practicing Oneness. "I used to come home mentally exhausted, my brain still at the office, half-listening to my daughter while checking emails. Now I set it all down when I walk through the door. I ask questions, and my daughter actually wants to answer them. We're closer than we have been in years."

These changes don't require conscious effort or any specific strategy. They emerge organically as the practice clears the mud from your mind, enabling you to connect deeply with those you love.

Transforming Workplace Dynamics

The workplace often presents unique challenges when it comes to maintaining our presence and balance. Deadlines, conflicting priorities, office politics, and the constant pressure to perform can trigger our most reactive patterns. Yet here too, Oneness can create remarkable shifts.

Joanne, who leads a design team at an ad agency, shared how her practice transformed her leadership approach. "I used to pride myself on my intensity—driving my team hard, always pushing for better results. After practicing Oneness for about a year, I realized I was creating unnecessary stress for everyone, including myself."

"Now, I bring the same quality of centered awareness to meetings that I cultivate in my Oneness practice," Joanne continued. "I listen more deeply. I don't react immediately to challenges or criticism. I've found that I can be more effective by not creating a storm of anxiety around me."

What's particularly interesting is how these individual changes can impact entire systems. Joanne noted that her team's dynamics shifted dramatically in response to her change in leadership style. "Turnover dropped. Creativity increased. People started collaborating more effectively," she said. "All because I changed how I showed up."

Organizations don't change through policies or restructuring alone. They change when the people within them transform their way of being.

Community Resonance

Even beyond families and workplaces, Oneness can create subtle yet powerful shifts in how we engage with our broader communities. The heightened awareness and reduced reactivity cultivated through practice naturally extend to our interactions with neighbors, service workers, and total strangers.

When you practice regularly, you start noticing how your energy affects others. Stand in line at the grocery store with anxiety and impatience, and watch how people around you tighten up. Stand with the same quality of presence you cultivate in Oneness practice, and the entire atmosphere shifts.

Our sensitivity to others increases. We begin to recognize that we're constantly participating in an energy exchange with everyone around us, either contributing to collective tension or helping to dissolve it.

Several studies on what researchers call "emotional contagion" confirm this phenomenon. Our nervous systems are constantly reading and responding to the emotional states of those around us, often below the level of our conscious awareness. By cultivating stability, ease, and presence through Oneness, we make a tangible contribution to our social environments.

Global Implications

At a time when societies worldwide face unprecedented challenges—environmental crises, political polarization, economic uncertainty—practices that foster awareness, compassion, and reduced reactivity have never been more essential.

Luckily, there is growing recognition of this need. Many major corporations now offer mindfulness programs to their employees. More and more schools are incorporating contemplative practices into their curricula. Healthcare systems increasingly integrate meditation into treatment protocols. Even military and law enforcement organizations have begun exploring these approaches.

What all these initiatives share is the recognition that our external challenges cannot be effectively addressed without inner transformation. As Grandmaster Yu observes, "Solving the world's problems begins with healing ourselves."

Oneness practice offers a particularly direct path to this healing. It doesn't require any superior physical or mental capabilities. It doesn't demand that you adhere to any specific belief system or adopt a new identity. It doesn't necessitate spending thousands of dollars on equipment, supplements, or training. Its simplicity makes it accessible across cultural and philosophical differences, allowing for widespread adoption without triggering resistance.

During these globally chaotic times, each person who commits to Oneness becomes a heart beating with clarity and peace. Each relationship transformed creates a small island of sanity and connection. Each workplace and community influenced by practitioners becomes a model, offering new ways of being together.

THE RIPPLE EFFECT

These ripples extend outward, intersecting with other movements and contributing to greater awareness and compassion. Oneness helps generate profound social transformation—not through force or persuasion, but through the natural influence of embodied presence.

By healing ourselves, we help heal our world. By finding our center, we help others find theirs. By embodying Oneness, we invite our family, friends, neighbors, coworkers and even perfect strangers into the same realm of peaceful possibility.

Chapter 24

100 Million Strong

Together, we have the power to spark a global movement offering people greater health, happiness, and compassion.

Every time I witness friends and family members experience life-changing transformations thanks to Oneness, and every time I hear the testimonials of students whose lives have been forever altered, I feel a renewed sense of purpose. These stories nurture my spirit again and again.

I was once hopeless. Like so many of you, I searched for answers in modern medicine and traditional Chinese medicine, but found none. I traveled many roads before discovering Oneness. And from the moment I set foot down this path, I found relief.

In this very moment, you may feel like I did then: On the brink of insanity, searching everywhere for relief, desperate for healing. Oneness healed me when nothing else could. That is why it has become my mission to share this powerful practice with you.

You are fortunate to have discovered this book. I sincerely hope to meet you in person one day soon. Meanwhile, please don't let the knowledge I have shared here stay only with you alone. Pass it along to someone you care about, someone who is suffering and in need of this life-changing practice.

ONENESS

Join me. Together, we have the power to spark a global movement offering people greater health, happiness, and compassion. Together, we can be 100 million strong.

Epilogue

True Peace

True peace
is not escaping the noise—
but letting it dissolve into music
that nourishes you.

True peace
is not silencing anger—
but resting in a stillness so deep,
anger no longer arises.

True peace
is smiling with the sky—
whether the sun warms your skin,
clouds blur your path,
or storms shake the air.

True peace
is showing love and empathy to those who test you,
those who annoy, resent, or try to harm—
and somehow, still wishing them peace.

True peace
is walking through the world in quiet awe,
grateful for the trees, the wind, the birds, the coyotes,

even the insects beneath your feet—
each one belonging, each one enough.

True peace
is remembering with gratitude—
not only those who stood by you
or pushed you to grow—
but also those who weren't kind,
the struggles and setbacks,
the pain and the pressure.
They didn't just pass through your life.
They shaped it.
They helped you become
exactly who you are.

True peace
is feeling that
everything is exactly as it should be.

Why I Refused to Add Pictures

(My Answer to a 3-Star Review)

A reader gave the book a 3-star review because it does not include any pictures or diagrams of the postures.

Why? The short answer is: This was a deliberate choice that I made for two reasons: 1) The posture looks slightly different for each person, and 2) The real secret of Oneness begins where the posture ends.

TLDR: A more complete answer below.

Dear Friend,

Oneness is so effective, yet it is not without challenges. The greatest challenges do not come from the practice itself, but from our human tendencies—our habits of striving, of trying harder, of believing that more effort or more complexity must be the answer. From childhood, our education has trained us to "do more, work harder, aim higher." **Oneness allows us to walk in the opposite direction: to let go, to do less, to simply be.**

This 3-star review gives me a chance to explain more clearly. Each time I try to explain, I notice that others begin to understand more deeply. And in truth, I also understand more myself.

This reader wrote that while they enjoyed the flow, they wished the book included pictures of the postures—saying they would have given 5 stars if illustrations were present. They also mentioned familiar names from other traditions such as "holding the balloon," "holding the tree," and "standing stake."

I deeply appreciate this comment because it points to something important. In the book, I explained briefly why I chose not to include pictures, but here I want to share the fuller reason.

Oneness is translated from the Chinese *Dacheng Lichan*. Its essence is simple yet profound: **non-doing, non-attaching, and being present.**

When Grandmaster Wang Xiangzhai, the founder of Dacheng Quan, first revealed this secret standing practice—known in Chinese as *Zhan Zhuang*—to the public in the 1950s, countless people benefitted. But he also gave a warning: *"While I am alive, there is only one practice. After I pass away, there will be hundreds."* His point was not to discourage practice, but to remind us that human nature often adds layers of complexity and distraction to something that is meant to be simple and direct.

Today, *Zhan Zhuang* and "standing practice" have become popular terms in China. Many people practice under those names, and these approaches may still bring benefit. But as Grandmaster Wang predicted, most versions emphasize posture details or external forms, and in doing so, sometimes overlook the deeper principle of **non-doing and letting go.**

The true goal of this practice is life transformation—not simply healing, not merely happiness, and not even mastery of Kung Fu. All of these are natural byproducts, but not the destination.

To preserve the essence, the second-generation Grandmaster Wang Xuanjie began using the term *Lichan*, emphasizing non-doing and non-attaching. Later, my teacher Grandmaster Yu Hongkun officially named it *Dacheng Lichan*. This is the tradition we call Oneness today. It is not about claiming superiority, but about safeguarding a path that remains faithful to its roots—direct, simple, and transformative.

Grandmaster Yu has authored seven books on this practice. None contain a single picture of the standing posture. I once asked him why. He told me:

"The design of our posture is so genius—it allows people to stand effortlessly in a way no other posture can. The posture matters, but it is only the beginning. Once the body is aligned, the real practice begins: being one with nature and simply enjoying. If I show my own posture, people will try to copy it. But everyone is different. If they focus only on getting the shape right, they will keep trying to look the same as me. The key teaching is not to reproduce the *same* posture, but to find the *right* posture—one that allows the body to align and stand effortlessly. Everyone's right posture will be different. That is why we try to avoid our students rigidly copying any image of the posture. The posture is a tool, not the destination. Its purpose is to help you stand effortlessly so you can truly connect with nature—effortless not only in the body but in the mind as well. If you attach to anything, either body or mind, it is no longer effortless. You are still trying, still striving."

This is why in Oneness you will not find names like "holding the balloon" or "holding the tree." Those belong to other systems. Our approach is different—not because we reject others, but because we emphasize what we believe is most essential: helping each person discover their own natural alignment, free from rigid imitation.

In our modern world, people already live with endless striving, desire, and attachment—the very causes of much chronic illness and mental suffering. Our minds are like muddy water, constantly stirred. Oneness helps the mud settle until the water becomes clear.

I know this path may feel unusual at first, because it asks us to do the opposite of what most of the world encourages. But as my teacher reminded me:

"LD, please don't compromise to appeal to trends. You may not find another practice as effective, as direct, as simple—for true life transformation."

That is why there are no pictures in this book. Not because posture doesn't matter, but because what lies beyond posture matters far more.

Please:

To help others discover Oneness, **leave a review**. Your words make it possible for more people to see this work—and each question or comment is also a chance for me to explain more clearly. Together, we can let Oneness reach and help 100 million people for life transformation in the most authentic way.

We're preparing courses and training, so people everywhere can practice Oneness and experience true life transformation for themselves.

Thank you for walking this path with me. Together, let's allow Oneness to reach the hearts of millions.

How to Stay in Touch

Thank you from the bottom of my heart for reading this book. Please do share it.

I believe that Oneness has the power to improve our lives on every level, and to profoundly impact the future of humanity. If you want to dive deeper into Oneness and even help us build it into a movement, I invite you to connect!

Subscribe to the free Oneness Institute newsletter to receive inspiration and practice suggestions. You'll also be first to hear about our affordable in-person training sessions.

Visit onenessinstitute.org/newsletter or simply scan the QR code below:

HELP OTHERS DISCOVER ONENESS

I spent more than 10 years searching before I finally discovered Oneness. Today, many people are still suffering from mental or physical challenges without finding a solution.

By leaving a review, you can help spread this information so others can discover Oneness much sooner, without the years of struggle I endured.

Your feedback not only supports me as an author, but also guides those who are still searching for healing and clarity.

Thank you from the bottom of my heart.

ABOUT THE AUTHORS

LD Chen

LD "William" Chen is an entrepreneur whose experience healing his mind and body through Oneness turned him into an avid teacher and champion of the ancient practice. A disciple of Oneness Grandmaster Yu Hongkun and a fourth-generation practitioner of Dacheng Quan, LD serves as the Head Coach of the Oneness Institute for America and Europe.

Having suffered throughout his youth in China from an array of debilitating illnesses including a heart attack, asthma, liver disease, chronic back pain, leg numbness, burnout and anxiety, LD spent his first decades of life on a quest for healing. In spite of enjoying all the outward trappings of success as a husband and father who built a successful multimillion-dollar clothing company from the ground up, he found himself in a state of despair. After a heart attack at age 32, he visited countless doctors looking for medical solutions. He also exercised daily and practiced Tai Chi. Nothing worked.

It was only when he discovered Oneness that LD's life transformed. The complete healing of mind and body that he experienced as a direct result of this simple yet powerful ancient wellness practice gave him a renewed sense of vitality and ignited his life purpose.

Under the guidance of Grandmaster Yu Hongkun—the author of seven books, teacher of thousands of practitioners, and sensei to many Oneness instructors—LD began teaching

Oneness to other people. He witnessed them experiencing transformations as profound as his. As a result, he became determined to help share the practice as widely as possible.

After immigrating to the U.S. with his family, LD enrolled in the Executive MBA program at the NYU Stern School of Business in 2020. Now, he is on a mission to introduce 100 million Westerners to Oneness, so that they might heal their physical ailments, elevate their mental health, and bring more peace and happiness to the world.

MeiMei Fox

Born in Hong Kong to an American diplomat and his wife, MeiMei picked up her Chinese name, which means "little sister," at age six months from her elder brother and their Mandarin-speaking nanny. A fanatical reader and lifelong writer, she has worked as a professional author, freelance editor, journalist, ghostwriter, and book coach for nearly three decades.

MeiMei is the founder and CEO of Your Bestselling Book, a company that provides a la carte writing and publishing support through services including a highly-acclaimed live 8-week course taught live in cohort with other thought leaders, as well as ghostwriting, one-on-one book coaching, and an online community platform, The Story Cure.

For nearly a decade, MeiMei was a paid contributor to *Forbes*. Her writing has also appeared in *The New York Times, Self, Stanford* magazine, *The Huffington Post*, and other esteemed publications. Two of her poems were selected for publication in compilations. Two books she co-authored were *New York Times* bestsellers, and two were selected for Oprah's Book List.

MeiMei earned a BA and MS in Psychology Phi Beta Kappa with Honors and Distinction from Stanford University, and an MA in Counseling Psychology from Pacifica Graduate Institute. She is a passionate yoga practitioner and enjoys a consistent meditation practice. She serves as Chair of the Board for HOPE

Foundation USA, an international NGO supporting vulnerable children and adults in Kolkata, India. Currently, she resides in Honolulu, Hawaii, with her husband Kiran Ramchandran and their twin boys.

www.ingramcontent.com/pod-product-compliance
Lightning Source LLC
Chambersburg PA
CBHW071259130626
46556CB00003B/1385